HOW TO "ACE" THE PHYSICIAN ASSISTANT SCHOOL INTERVIEW

From the author of the best-selling book,
The Ultimate Guide to Getting Into Physician Assistant School

Andrew J. Rodican, PA-C

ISBN: 0615480721
ISBN-13: 9780615480725
LCCN: 2011906514

Contents

Introduction

If you are reading this book, either you or someone you know wants to be a physician assistant (PA). And why not?

In 2009, *U.S. News & World Report* ranked the PA profession in the "top 30" careers for job satisfaction, prestige, job market outlook, and salary. The U.S. Labor Bureau finds it to be the third fastest growing profession in the country.

That's the good news!

The bad news is that the competition for getting into PA school is fierce. And the most qualified applicant isn't necessarily the one who gets accepted. The applicant who sells him- or herself most effectively is the one who gets accepted.

Your chances of getting into the PA school of your choice average 5 to 9 percent based on current statistics. For example, Baylor College of Medicine's PA program receives over seven hundred applications per year. One hundred applicants are interviewed, and only thirty-five applicants are accepted, which equates to 5 percent of total applicants achieving success.

Even if you meet or exceed all of the prerequisites, write a killer essay, and get invited to the interview, you still need to deliver the performance of your life in the interview if you're going to be selected.

This book will help you deliver that performance. There is a common misperception that there is no real way to prepare for an interview. Nothing could be further from the truth. No matter what type of interview you have, whether it is relaxed or formal being prepared is the one key to your success.

Before we get to the details of how to have a successful interview, you will need a little context on the profession and a bit more information about the process so that you can accomplish your goal: a spot in the PA program of your choice!

THE HISTORY OF THE PA PROFESSION

The physician assistant profession dates back to the 1960s, when there was a shortage and uneven geographic distribution of primary-care physicians in the United States. In an attempt to ease the problems associated with this shortage, Dr. Eugene Stead of Duke University Medical Center decided to start a physician assistant training program and assembled an inaugural class. This class was composed of former U.S.

Navy hospital corpsman and U.S. Army combat medics, who had received considerable medical training during their military service.

This class graduated on October 6, 1967, a date that is now considered to be the official anniversary date of the PA profession. October 6–11 has been designated National Physician Assistant Week in honor of this class.

During the 1970s, the U. S. Army was the primary user of physician assistants. The army was losing many physicians to civilian practice and quickly saw the benefit of PAs. In 1971, Congress authorized the training of four hundred army PAs. The first army class graduated in July of 1973. The other services quickly followed the army's lead and established their own programs.

From that first class of four PAs at Duke University Medical Center, the PA profession grew rapidly and currently has over 88,000 PAs eligible to practice. The Bureau of Labor Statistics projects that there will be demand for 150,000 physician assistants by the year 2020. And it is likely that the demand will continue to increase long after 2020.

WHO THEY ARE AND WHAT THEY CAN PRACTICE

Just over 65 percent of practicing physician assistants are female. The average age for a PA student is twenty-seven. Practice options are varied, and PAs may practice in many areas including primary care, surgical specialties, emergency medicine, internal medicine, pediatrics, and other specialty areas. Physician assistants can work for others (in clinics and hospitals) or even for themselves (private practice with other health-care professionals working for them).

IT'S HARDER THAN YOU THINK

While this information isn't meant to discourage you, it is important you know that getting into physician assistant school is harder than you may think.

The University of Iowa was ranked number one in physician assistant programs by *U. S. News and World Report*. In 2010, they accepted 25 of 630 applicants.

The truth is getting into medical school may be easier than getting into physician assistant school, so it is important to avoid mistakes. Your chance of acceptance dramatically decreases after you have been rejected once. You have to do it right the first time!

THE FIVE MAJOR MISTAKES APPLICANTS MAKE WHEN CONSIDERING PA SCHOOL

Before you apply to a program, it is important to consider the ramifications of going to PA school. I have found five major mistakes candidates make as they consider PA school.

Mistake No. 1: Giving in to Financial Fears

Physician assistant school is expensive. It is also a lot of work and requires time spent studying and in clinical rotations. Candidates are often unsure whether or not to quit a current job. So while careful consideration is important, you shouldn't let financial fears get in the way of making the best decisions for you.

Most programs display costs for PA school on their Web site. You can expect to spend over $30,000 per year on school, but PAs earn anywhere between the high $70,000s and $110,000 per year. From these numbers, you can calculate your return on investment (e.g. two years with no salary and tuition costs compared to earning potential when you get out).

Additionally, ask yourself the following questions:

1.   Can I afford to become a PA?
2.   Can I afford not to become a PA?
3.   Where will I be in five years (as a PA or not)?
4.   Can I afford to give up my current job while I attend school?
5.   Is my current employment secure?

Answering these questions honestly will provide you with the insight you need to make the best decisions for you and your family and avoid making a mistake because of financial fears.

Mistake No. 2: Having Mistaken Motivations

Passion is the rocket fuel that drives the car to success. In order to sacrifice what is needed to be successful in physician assistant school and as a physician assistant, you need to be sure that you want to be a PA. If you are serious and passionate about and committed to becoming a PA, you will be successful. Without these factors, you are just another fish in the ocean.

Passion comes from the Latin word, *passio,* meaning "to suffer." In other words, in order to achieve your goal and become a PA, you must be willing to sacrifice. To be willing to suffer, you must be motivated and have a clear goal.

Researchers who have studied successful people have determined that they accomplished their goals by doing three things. First, they wrote their goals on paper. The mere act of writing them out—articulating them on paper—reinforced the goal. Second, they held themselves accountable for their goals. Finally, they made a commitment to themselves and others to accomplish those goals.

Mistake No. 3: Making Application Blunders

The single biggest mistake applicants make during the application process is that they don't pay strict enough attention to the details. Being successful as a PA requires attention to detail because you are dealing with patients. A careless mistake can mean serious injury or death.

Mistakes in your application, such as typos, grammatical errors, and failure to follow directions, will communicate to the committee that you don't attend to details. A careless application means a careless professional.

Recommendations can also cause problems in the application process. When thinking about recommendations, you should consider many things.

First, applicants often assume that a letter of recommendation from a prestigious physician or scholar improves their chances of being accepted into PA school. That is not necessarily true, especially if that person doesn't know you well—which is often the case. You are far better off getting a letter from someone who knows you well and can speak about you from personal experience. These people can give specific examples of why they think you will be a good candidate for PA school and the profession.

Second, many recommenders write as if the applicant is applying for a job. Instead, they should focus on you as a potential student, not employee. Also consider this when you select your recommender: a person who can recommend you for a job may not be the same person you would like to have recommend you for PA school. The job reference will likely be geared toward individual productivity and performance, whereas the PA school reference should be geared more toward personal skills and how you fit in as a team player.

Third, remember that your letter is not a character reference. Someone you know from church or your grandmother who has had a lot of medical care can attest to your many good qualities but will not be very helpful at assessing your candidacy to PA school.

Finally, try to pick someone who can be as unbiased as possible. Though the chair of surgery in a large medical center in your hometown is a friend of the family and knows you well, he or she may still not be a good reference if the committee believes that this person is unable to be objective about you.

Mistake No. 4: Falling into Common Essay Pitfalls

This is important: applicants who fail to use the personal statement to frame their candidacy are making a serious mistake.

Your personal statement may be the single most important piece of writing you will do in your medical career. Do not use this valuable real estate to reiterate the contents of your résumé. Use this statement to make a personal connection with the reader and create a desire in that person to meet you in person.

The essay can be your ticket to the interview; however, it can also be the kiss of death!

Presentation is important. Badly written essays give a negative impression and may even alienate the admissions officers who read them. Essays are the most time-consuming part of the admissions process for the admissions officers, and reading a poorly written essay can be a painful experience for the officer. If he or she feels pain reading your essay, you will not be invited in for an interview.

Before you begin writing, you should assess your audience. The readers will be looking for your motivation for being a PA, the effectiveness of your communication skills, evidence of soft skills (people skills), and the extent to which you are genuine.

In order to communicate this to them, you must first get their attention and draw them into your essay. You must also keep them interested. Use stories and give examples to draw them in and keep them interested. Your stories will tell them who you are and why you are unique.

Here are some tips for essay construction and writing:

I.   Start with the end in mind—As you write, remember your end goal. Your goal is to stand out from the crowd. A killer essay will make you stand out from the crowd. Think about how you can do that before you begin writing.

2. Style—Have someone read your essay (you would be surprised how many essays I have read where I thought: *This applicant obviously did not have anyone read this before sending it in.*)

3. Grammar—Proofread for grammatical errors. If you aren't comfortable doing this, get some help from someone who is.

4. Content—Check your content. Are you saying something important? Are you making an emotional connection with the readers? Are you answering the question(s) they are asking?

5. Brevity—Review each sentence and ask: Can I say this in fewer words? Have I already said this?

6. Clichés—Be original and unique. After 9/11, many applicants said they wanted to be a PA because the events of that day moved them to make a difference. I wouldn't be surprised if this year's applicants mention the BP oil spill or health-care reform.

7. Big words—You don't need to use big words to communicate effectively. Using longer, fancier words only tells the readers that you know how to use a thesaurus.

8. Hot topics—Avoid hot topics—especially if you intend to get on your soapbox and rant. Readers want to know about you, not about the political issues about which you are concerned.

A well-written essay will pass the "easy and enjoyable to read" test and will stimulate the readers to want to get to know you better. Keep that in mind as you write your essay, and you will avoid many of these essay pitfalls.

Mistake No. 5: Getting All the Way to the Interview and Missing the Mark

The purpose of this book is to help you avoid this mistake. As was mentioned above, preparation is key. There are some important things to think about first.

You need to know about current events and relative topics, such as health-care reform, managed care, and the role of the PA in the future. You must also know who will be conducting the interview—an individual or a group—or if it will be a casual roundtable interview and how to handle those dynamics. You need to know the scoring criteria, and finally and most important, you must know the answers to the questions you will be asked! I will discuss all of these important factors in the following chapters.

Understanding the Physician Assistant School Interview

1

The PA school interview will be unlike many of the interviews you have experienced in the past. In order to perform well, you will need to have a thorough understanding of the scoring criteria, the different types of interviews, and the interview questions you are likely to be asked. Armed with this knowledge, you will be more confident and relaxed when it is your turn to "stand tall."

The Interview Process

Knowing what to expect at the interview will help you be more prepared, relieve your anxiety, and enable you to concentrate solely on giving the performance of your life. Although interview protocols vary from program to program, you should be aware of some of the most frequent scenarios.

Upon arriving at the interview, applicants usually proceed to a common area where they will have a chance to meet and socialize with the other candidates. Once all candidates are present, one or more of the PA program's staff will address the group. They will give you a schedule for the day and some general information about the program. The admissions officer and the financial aid officer might also brief the group. Some programs will have you either write a short essay or answer a set of ethical questions. After you have completed all of these preliminaries, the actual interviewing process begins.

There are typically three types of interviews: the individual interview, the group interview, and the student interview.

I. The individual interview—One of the PA program faculty usually conducts these interviews. The interviewer could be the medical director, the dean of the program, the associate dean, or the clinical coordinator. The objective of having this type of interview is to determine if the applicant's answers are consistent with the answers given in the other interviews that day and to see if he or she would be a good "fit" for the program.

2. The group interview—Prior graduates of the PA program or professors who teach in the program generally handle group interviews. The purpose of this interview is to see how the candidates conduct themselves under stress, to evaluate their communication skills, and to see how well they handle tough interview questions.

3. The student interview—First- and second-year PA students run the student interviews. These students want to know if the candidate is a team player, if the candidate has worked as hard as they have to get there, and if he or she has the right "attitude." Caution: *do not take this interview lightly.*

SCORING YOUR INTERVIEW

At the completion of each interview, the committee members give you an overall score. At the end of the day, the committee meets to debate your scores and provide you with a final grade.

Following is a list of the scoring criteria and key factors most PA program admissions committees use to judge you:

1. Cognitive and verbal ability
   a. Can you think a problem through and respond appropriately?
   b. Can you articulate your ideas in a logical sequence?
   c. Are you perceptive about others?
   d. Are you organized?
   e. Do you have good time-management skills?
   f. Do you understand and grasp the intensity of the PA program?

2. Motivation to become a PA
   a. Are you strongly motivated or just testing the water?
   b. Are you interested in patients or the "science" of medicine?
   c. Do you consider PA school to be a stepping-stone to medical school?
   d. Have you completed all of your prerequisites?
   e. Do you have the required medical experience?

     f.   Have you shadowed any PAs?

3. Understanding of the PA profession
    a.   Do you know what PA practice entails?
    b.   Have you worked with any PAs?
    c.   What is your attitude toward nurses?
    d.   Do you understand the dependent nature of the profession?
    e.   Do you understand the autonomous nature of the profession?
    f.   Do you know the history of the PA profession?

4. Interpersonal skills and behavior
    a.   Do you work collaboratively?
    b.   Do your colleagues and co-workers respect you?
    c.   Are you domineering or a team player?
    d.   Are you compassionate?
    e.   Are you empathetic?
    f.   Are you well groomed?

5. Ability to handle stress
    a.   Can you be clear, concise, and relaxed at the interview?
    b.   What does stress represent to you?
    c.   Do you remain poised and relatively calm in the face of stressful situations?
    d.   Do you have a sense of humor?
    e.   Can you think on your feet?

6. Personal characteristics
    a.   Are you thoughtful and innovative?
    b.   Are the facts you convey in the interview consistent with your experience?
    c.   Are you mature?
    d.   Are you driven?
    e.   Do you have passion?
    f.   Are you a motivator?

Later in the book, you will learn about the specific interview questions and answers relative to the above scoring criteria. But first, you have to convince one very important person that you should be admitted to PA school. Who is that person? You! Preparation is the key to silencing your "inner critic."

WHAT DO YOU HAVE TO OFFER?

Some interviewers will look to your knowledge and experience to score you the highest. Others may look for specific skills you possess that are transferable.

Knowledge-Based Skills

You must first identify your own knowledge-based skills. Here are some examples. Are you:

- Organized
- Calm
- An effective communicator
- A team player
- A leader
- Good with time management
- A counselor

Do you have:

- A science background
- A medical background
- A military background
- Experience working in underserved areas

Transferable Skills

Transferable skills are important when you don't have medical experience, but you've worked in several positions that required many of the skills needed to become a PA. These skills can come in handy when writing your essay or when interviewing.

Keep in mind that most PA programs are not looking to fill a class with "clones"; your unique experiences may be just what they need to round out an incoming class.

Some examples of transferable skills include: communication skills; organizational skills; leadership skills; teaching, coaching, or customer service skills; problem-solving and conflict resolution skills; etc.

Make your own list of transferable skills:

- _Conflict resolution skills_
- _customer service_
- _communication_
- _organization_
- _____

Personal Traits

Personal traits are what make you unique. You cannot teach these skills. You either have them, or you don't. My favorite is passion! Other examples of personal traits include: high energy, cooperative style, calmness, flexibility (go with the flow), empathy, patience, and humor.

Make your own list of personal traits:

- _calm_
- _flexible_
- _ambitious_
- _kind_
- _accountable_

Exercise: The Three P's

Now that you have identified some of your skills, it's time to lay them out on paper. Divide a piece of paper into three columns and label them with the headings "Education and Previous Experience," "Portable Skills," and "Personality Traits." Like the three P's of marketing, this will be your PA school marketing tool.

EDUCATION AND PREVIOUS EXPERIENCE

(Examples: X-ray technician, medical assistant, retail store manager, customer service representative)

- _mental health tech_

- _____
- _____
- _____
- _____

PORTABLE/TRANSFERABLE SKILLS

(Examples: skills related to customer relations, communications, time management, organization, analysis)

- Customer relations
- communication skills
- Conflict resolution
- _____
- _____

PERSONALITY TRAITS

(Examples: passionate, motivated, self-starter, friendly, positive, industrious)

- Cooperative
- Calm
- Flexibility
- patience
- Motivated

When you're done, check each list to see a summary of the accomplishments, skills, and traits that you have to offer.

The next step is to plan your strategy to show off these traits in the stories you'll tell at your interview. Use these traits and stories to convince the committee that you meet the criteria they're looking for.

Remember, you need to sell yourself to the admissions committee and give them enough reasons to make the decision to select you an easy one. Here are some strong suggestions to make that happen:

1)   Write out your educational/work summary and goals:

Make a list of your core values and goals. Include short-range goals (one year or less), medium-range goals (two to five years), and long-range goals (five years or more).

2)   Develop your unique selling proposition (USP):

You are going to be interviewing with several other strong applicants. You will need to stand out in the crowd (in a positive way) if you are going to claim your seat in next year's class. What will make you more unique, valuable, and visible at the interview? A strong USP.

Developing a unique selling proposition or "USP" will dramatically increase the likelihood of positioning yourself as the best applicant.

The USP will do three things for you. It will:

a.   Show how you are unique—It clearly sets you apart from your competition, positioning you as the more logical choice.

b.   Sell you—It persuades the committee to choose you over anyone else.

c.   Proposes you—It is a proposal or offer that suggests you for acceptance.

Getting into PA school is a challenging task at best. You must have a USP that "cuts through the clutter," separates you from the competition, and positions you as the best choice…the *only* choice.

Building your USP takes some effort, but it is absolutely worth it because of the added advantage you'll have in the interview. A powerful USP will make your job of selling yourself to the admissions committee much easier, enabling you to increase your odds of getting accepted.

An effective USP alleviates the "pain" experienced by the admissions committee when they try to figure out which applicants are the best "fit" for their program.

The admissions committee has multiple excellent applicants to choose from, and it's difficult at times to know which applicants to select. When the committee asks you why they should select you, realize that they are not trying to intimidate you; rather, they are asking for your help. So help them out!

Here is a good example of a winning USP:

I have five years of hands-on medical experience, excellent communication and interpersonal skills, a strong ability to handle stress, and a thorough understanding of the PA profession, and I have the test scores and GRE to demonstrate my ability to handle a rigorous didactic program. I also have the ability to lead or be a team player, depending on the circumstances. Invest in me, and you can rest assured that you've made the right decision.

What is your USP?

WHAT ARE THE MOST IMPORTANT CHARACTERISTICS IN A PA?

If you want to make a strong case for your candidacy, you first need to understand the characteristics that make a good physician assistant and then identify how your specific background matches up with these characteristics.

As mentioned already, you will be evaluated in five specific areas when you apply to a PA program:

1. Passion
2. Academic ability and test scores
3. Medical experience
4. Understanding of the PA profession
5. Maturity

Passion

Passion cannot be quantified. Passion, or the lack thereof, can make or break your chances of getting accepted to PA school. Applicants can demonstrate passion by having a thorough understanding of the PA profession and by having accomplished prerequisites "above and beyond" the average applicant.

EXERCISE:

List five things you've done to demonstrate your passion to become a PA. Examples might include shadowing experiences, medical experience, extra coursework to raise your GPA, etc.:

1. _Completing prerequisite coursework +_
2. _Shadowing PAs (ortho + family)_
3. _Mental health tech_
4. _CNA/PCT_
5. _Attended open house/current journal reading_

Academic Ability and Test Scores

Approximately 83 percent of PA school applicants have a bachelor's degree and approximately 50 percent of PA school applicants have a degree in biology.

Exercise: Fill in the following chart with your data.

	Average Stats from Emory Number applicants: 857 Candidates interviewed: 177	Your Numbers
Undergraduate GPA	3.3	3.79
Natural Sciences GPA	3.2	3.75
GRE Verbal	520	
GRE Quantitative	610	
GRE Analytical	4.5	
Healthcare Experience (hrs)	5900	1500

Medical Experience

More than three-quarters (79 percent) of PA school applicants report having worked in a health-care field, either part-time or full-time, prior to enrolling in PA school. Only 27 percent of applicants worked less than one year or not at all in a health-care field (regardless of direct patient contact), while 10 percent worked more than nine years in a health-care field. Thirty-five percent of applicants worked less than one year or not at all in a health-care field with direct patient contact.[1]

Overall, 18 percent of PA school applicants previously worked as a medical assistant, 17 percent worked as an EMT/paramedic, 9 percent worked as a phlebotomist, 8 percent worked as an emergency room technician, 7 percent worked in medical reception/records, 8 percent worked as a nurse, and 6 percent worked as an athletic trainer.

Forty percent of applicants reported "other" as a previous health-care field of employment.

Understanding of the PA Profession

Eighty-nine percent of respondents knew at least one PA prior to applying to PA school. If you don't know a PA, make sure you create an opportunity to meet one.

Here are some questions that relate to your understanding of the profession, which you should consider before you apply:

1. Are you a member of the American Academy of Physician Assistants (AAPA)?
2. Are you a member of your state (constituent) chapter of the AAPA?
3. Have you shadowed at least four PAs?
4. How many PAs do you know?

Maturity

Maturity is another one of those areas that you can't quantify. You should have a basic understanding of what maturity means to the admissions committee.

Here are some questions they will be thinking about:

1. Can you be empathetic, yet assertive?
2. Can you handle stress under fire?
3. Will you know when to call for help?

---

[1]   Note: respondents were permitted to indicate multiple previous health-care fields; thus, the sum of all fields exceeds 100 percent.

4. Do you exhibit good judgment?
5. Can you make quick decisions?
6. Are you a self-starter?
7. Will you require constant supervision?

EXERCISE

a. Write down the dictionary definitions of *empathetic* and *assertive*:

Empathetic: _Showing ready comprehension of others' states_

Assertive: _confident and direct_

b) Describe a situation where you've had to be empathetic, yet assertive:

Patient becoming aggressive due to chronic back pain.

c) Describe a stressful situation that you were able to resolve:

Patient on home unit wouldn't take PRN
meds - was becoming combative. Was called to
unit. I acted as nothing was wrong and due to
positive rapport, patient complied.

d) Write down the dictionary definition of the word *judgment*.

Judgment: _____

e) Write down the dictionary definition of *autonomous*.

Autonomous: _____

Soft Skills

At this point, we should also discuss "soft skills." *Soft skills* is a sociological term relating to a person's cluster of personality traits, social graces, communication abilities, language competence, personal habits, friendliness, and optimism that characterize relationships with other people. Soft skills complement hard skills (grades and test scores) that are the occupational requirements of a job and many other activities.

Soft skills are as equally sought out by admissions committees as hard skills. Soft skills may actually be more important over the long term than hard skills. A physician assistant must have excellent interpersonal skills to be effective.

The admissions committee is going to look for proficiency in the following areas:

- Communication skills
- Conflict resolution and negotiation
- Personal effectiveness
- Creative problem solving
- Strategic thinking
- Teamwork
- Persuasion skills
- Listening skills

EXERCISE:

List four people skills at which you excel. Also, think of a story that demonstrates your use of that skill. Examples might include a time you worked collaboratively on a team to solve a problem, etc.

1. _empathy/empathic_
2. _compassionate_
3. _flexible/easy going_
4. _approachable_

DO YOUR HOMEWORK

The admissions committee will expect you to have a thorough understanding of the PA profession and their school. One of the major scoring criteria is passion. One definition of the word *passion* is boundless enthusiasm, and another definition is to sacrifice. If you have boundless enthusiasm and you've been willing to sacrifice, then surely you have spent a great deal of time doing your homework, correct? The chances are extremely high that you will be asked one or more of the following questions:

- When/how did the PA profession get its start?
- What are some of the issues facing PAs today?
- How will health-care reform affect PAs?
- What are some of the greatest challenges facing PAs today?
- What is the difference between a PA and a nurse practitioner?
- Why don't you want to become a nurse practitioner?
- Why do you want to attend our program?
- What do you know about the history of our program?
- Did you attend our open house?

Be sure to do your homework. You can find the answers to most of these questions in my book, *The Ultimate Guide to Getting into Physician Assistant School*[2] or on my Web site, www.AndrewRodican.com. However, there are many other resources available to you:

- American Academy of Physician Assistants (AAPA)—www.aapa.org
- Student Academy of the American Academy of Physician Assistants (SAAPA)—http://www.aapa.org/student-academy)
- Physician Assistant Education Association (PAEA)—http://www.paeaonline.org
- PA Programs Directory—http://www.paeaonline.org
- Each PA Program's Web site
- PA students
- PA Forum—www.physicianassistantforum.com
- Physician assistants in the community

Be sure to research the faculty at each PA program in which you receive an invitation to interview. Find out where they went to PA school, in which area of medicine they practice, and what their relationship is to the PA program.

Spend time practicing interpersonal skills and high-impact communication skills. I dedicate a full chapter to these areas in my book.

---

2   3rd Ed. McGraw-Hill. ISBN 978-0-07-163973-6, 2011

Also, have an understanding of the types of interviews that are conducted at each school (individual interview, group interview, student interview, and roundtable interviews).

Finally, learn what interview questions you are most likely to be asked and practice your answers.

FINDING THE BEST "FIT"

One significant purpose of the PA school interview is to determine if the school is a good "fit" for your objectives. With over 144 PA programs in the United States at the time of this writing, applicants should, at the very least, inquire about the following at each interview:

- Are there any discrepancies with the program's first-time pass/fail rates on the NCCPA boards (if applicable)?
- What is the philosophy/focus of the program?
- What is the availability of clinical rotation sites?
- How is the quality of clinical rotation sites?
- Is there a cadaver lab?
- Who teaches the classes?
- What is the class size?

After all, you are the one paying for this educational experience. The only way to find out if you will be getting a good value for your investment is to inquire about the items listed above and anything else that you consider significant to making your decision.

The benefit of asking intelligent questions is threefold: 1) you will come across as an educated consumer; 2) you will feel more in control of the interview; and 3) you will gather enough information to make an informed decision on whether you should rule in or rule out the program.

THE FOUR TYPES OF INTERVIEW QUESTIONS

A strong PA school applicant will be prepared to answer the toughest interview questions. Here are four types of questions you will be asked:

1. Traditional
2. Behavioral
3. Ethical
4. Situational

In Chapter 3, I cover the toughest interview questions and answers for traditional questions. Traditional questions are some of the most commonly asked questions at the PA school interview.

In Chapter 4, I cover the newest type of interview questions—behavioral questions. Unlike traditional questions, you will be challenged to think on your feet and often "describe" a specific situation in which you had to deal with stress, a difficult situation with a co-worker, or a time when you had to utilize effective communication skills. The premise behind behavioral questions is that past behavior is likely to dictate future behavior, given a similar set of circumstances. Behavioral interviewing questions seek to understand how you will behave as a PA.

Chapter 5 deals with ethical questions. Ethical questions can make or break your interview. If you know the most common ethical questions, you will not have to be so anxious on interview day.

Chapter 6 addresses situational interviewing. Situational questions place you in a specific scenario in order to find out how you would react or to find out the answer to the question, "What would you do?"

THE "CASUAL" OR "ROUNDTABLE" INTERVIEW

Many PA programs use a type of interview that may seem innocuous at first glance but can be devastating if you underestimate its purpose. The casual or roundtable interview is a group interview; only the "group" consists of you, the other applicants, and one or two admissions committee members.

The reason that this type of interview is so stressful is that questions are thrown out to the group for anyone to answer. If you are at all shy or unprepared, you will be swallowed up by the competition. Additionally, if you become anxious during the interview, you will go into "fight-or-flight" mode, and your brain will shut down. (Later in the book, I will teach you a powerful technique to calm your anxiety in about thirty seconds.)

Once again, preparation is the key to success throughout the whole interview process. The more prepared you are, the less likely you are to panic. In the casual or roundtable interview, you will need to find a balance between being too passive and being too aggressive. The goal is to be assertive!

So what is the difference between passive, assertive, and aggressive? Here is a brief synopsis of each communication style:

Passive:	"You win; I lose."
Aggressive:	"I win; you lose."
Passive/Aggressive:	"I lose; you lose."
Assertive:	"You win; I win."

Keep these communication styles in mind when you interact with other applicants, the program staff, and the admissions committee members. The goal is to create a win-win scenario.

DEALING WITH ANXIETY

When you wake on the day of your interview, I can assure you that your heart will be racing, your breath will be shallow and rapid, and your mind will be a little foggy. Don't panic! What you're experiencing is healthy anxiety. Your body's physiology is acting appropriately. The challenge is to avoid panicking.

Think about this; when we are in panic mode, our brain shuts down. It is not exactly a time to do your taxes! So if you want to be able to think clearly, particularly on the day of your interview, you need to control your physiology.

If you are not prepared, your plan is to "wing it." This plan is going to cause a lot of anxiety, and you will be in the fight-or-flight mode throughout the entire interview process. When you are in fight-or-flight mode, your physiology changes as follows:

1. Your heart rate increases
2. Your pupils dilate
3. Your breathing gets shallow
4. Your brain shuts down

So, if you're in this type of physiology, you won't be able to think of an answer. You'll appear nervous. You will not make the impression that you're hoping to make, and you'll likely receive a very low score on your interview.

Dr. Eva Selhub, a mind/body expert, resiliency coach, motivational speaker, and executive coach teaches a powerful technique used to instantly reduce a person's stress and anxiety level.

Her technique is the SHIELD® technique, and the acronym stands for:

Stop
Honor the feeling
Inhale
Exhale
Listen
Decide

Author of *The Love Response*,[3] Dr. Selhub promotes a simple philosophy:
At its best, stress motivates. At its worst, stress annihilates.
Good leaders motivate. Bad leaders annihilate.
The choice is yours to decide how stress will influence your leadership.[4]

If you find yourself in an anxiety-provoking or stressful situation (like the PA school interview), you can use the SHIELD® technique to instantly change your physiology. As a result, your breathing will slow down, your heart rate will decrease, your pupils will return to normal size, and you will be able to think much more clearly.

Here is how the technique works:

Once you feel your anxiety level becoming too high, *stop* what you are doing. Then, *honor the feeling*. Are you anxious, afraid, frustrated, angry, lonely, or tired? Next, *inhale* and *exhale*, ten times in a row. (When you breathe in, imagine filling an empty balloon in your belly with your breath. When you breathe out, imagine deflating the balloon.) Repeat the breaths ten times, and you will notice a soothing, calming effect. By this time, you're physiology is changing, and you will be able to think clearly and focus on the task at hand. So, *listen* to your mind and become aware of your thoughts and feelings. Finally, *decide* to do something different than ruminating, which is counterproductive.

You can repeat the above technique as many times as necessary to help you relax and focus.

SILENCING THE "INNER CRITIC"

In a variety of stressful situations, we become our own worst enemy. I can remember arriving for my interview at Yale and meeting all of my "competition." Everyone in the room had a master's degree, except for me. My inner critic came alive. "I'm never

---

3   Ballantine (2009).
4   For more information, check out Dr. Selhub's Web site: http://www.DrSelhub.com.

going to get in!" I was being very hard on myself and extremely judgmental. Negative self-talk only serves to perpetuate the anxiety and make things worse.

Here are some things your inner critic may shout at you on the day of your interview:

- "I should have prepared more."
- "Everyone here is more qualified than I am."
- "I'll never get accepted."
- "I'm a loser; I don't belong here."
- "I'm going to blow this interview."

Don't wait until your interview to address your inner critic. Here are some steps that you can take to deal with your inner critic weeks or months before your interview:

1. Monitor your thoughts.

Becoming aware of your inner critic's voice, if you will, is the first step. You can achieve this by simply being mindful of those thoughts. Just notice when and where the thoughts occur, and then write them down on a piece of paper or in a journal. You may become acutely aware of certain patterns in your thinking. Once you master being mindful and get the negative thoughts on paper, you can begin to silence the inner critic.

2. Notice your judgments.

Instead of making judgments, try describing your thoughts or feelings. For example, you may be having a conversation with a fellow student about a class you are both taking. You may really like the professor, and in the course of the conversation, you might say, "Professor Jones is a great teacher. Your classmate might not agree with you and say, "I think he's a terrible teacher." Both of you are making judgments and probably putting the other person on guard to defend his or her decision.

If you said instead, "I appreciate that Professor Jones always comes prepared to class. It makes it easier for me to stay focused." You are not being judgmental; you are simply describing the way you feel about him. Nobody can dispute that, not even your friend.

The point is that when we are being judgmental, especially of ourselves, we promote more intense feelings of negativity. And at the interview, we want to stay positive.

3. Challenge your automatic negative thoughts.

Feelings aren't facts! Once you practice mindfulness and become good at documenting your thoughts (judgments), it is time to challenge those negative thoughts with the facts. You may feel like you don't have what it takes to be accepted, but if you look at the facts, you may change your mind.

For example, if you were to review your CASPA application, you would see that you've worked hard to complete the requirements for PA school. The fact that you received an offer to interview means that you already beat out several hundred applicants to get the interview. So although you may certainly feel like you don't have what it takes to get accepted, the facts prove otherwise.

Try to challenge all of your negative thoughts with the facts. Chances are you will find that you are beating yourself up for no reason.

4. Practice, not perfection.

The goal of practicing mindfulness and keeping your judgments in check is to achieve awareness and make gradual changes. Becoming aware of the problem is the first step. However, if you are in denial about how your judgments and negative thoughts affect your mind-set, you will not be able to make any progress at all. It takes constant vigilance to achieve improvement with being mindful.

5. Reevaluate your values.

Make sure that whatever you are beating yourself up over is worth striving for. Some goals, like kindness, integrity, and being self-disciplined, enhance the meaning and quality of life, whereas others only feed into your sense of defectiveness. Some people think, *If I only went to a better school, I'd have more self-esteem.* But the way to increase self-esteem is to do estimable things.

TWENTY-FOUR HOURS AND COUNTING

The day before your interview, you may be thinking, *All of the work I've done to get into PA school will ride on my performance tomorrow.* And you know what? You're right. Depending on your preparation, you will either get accepted or get rejected.

Planning ahead will help you achieve your goal of getting accepted. If you have twenty-four hours to dedicate to planning prior to your interview, here are my recommendations:

1. Twenty-four hours before your interview, or about 8:00 a.m., drive from your hotel or your home to the exact location of your interview. Get a feel for the time you'll need the next day, the traffic flow, and the parking situation. You may even choose to go into the building to find the exact location of the interview.

2. During the drive home or back to the hotel, use visualization to "psych" yourself up for the next day. See yourself arriving and greeting the program staff and the other applicants in a relaxed and confident way.

3. The night before, get prepared. Review all the materials and exercises presented earlier in this chapter. Practice answering questions aloud to a "fake" interviewer or to yourself if that helps you prepare.

4. Get a good night's sleep.

5. Leave yourself plenty of time to get to the interview site. Plan to get there early so you can once again review your notes and get emotionally ready for the day.

6. Interview time: You have done all your preparation and homework. Relax and have fun. Remember that you are interviewing them as well to be certain that this program would be a good fit for you.

The Top Five Interview Mistakes

2

There is no room for mistakes on interview day.

Recently, I posted a poll question on the PA Forum[5] asking PA school admissions committee members: "What is the number-one mistake PA school applicants make at the interview?" The results were as follows:

The following list constitutes the top five mistakes (in ascending order:

1. Poor answers to interview questions   35 percent
2. Not being "likeable"   24 percent
3. Sense of entitlement based on résumé   20 percent
4. Not making an emotional connection   12 percent
5. Inappropriate dress/accessories   9 percent

Let's examine ways to make a favorable impression in each one of these areas.

MISTAKE #1: INABILITY TO EFFECTIVELY ANSWER INTERVIEW QUESTIONS

The number-one reason cited in my research for not recommending a candidate for a PA program is that he or she did not answer the interview questions effectively.

The rest of this book focuses on ways to ensure that you don't fall into this category. If you read the remainder of this book and do the exercises in it, you will have seriously increased your odds of getting into PA school because you will have prepared yourself for the most important part of the process: the interview!

---

5   http://www.physicianassistantforum.com/forums/forum.php

MISTAKE #2: NOT BEING LIKEABLE

All things being equal, committee members will select the applicant who comes across as the most likeable. As I have already mentioned, people base most decisions on emotions and support them with logic.

How to Increase Your Likeability

Here are some likeability skills–building steps to enhance your message and increase your likeability score:

1. Friendliness—Get yourself into the "zone" before walking into the interview. Have a friendly mind-set and communicate friendliness at all times. In my book, *The Ultimate Guide to Getting into Physician Assistant School*, I recommend that you practice answering interview answers with a tape recorder and play it back to listen to your tone. Is it friendly?

    A good tip is to practice smiling when talking to someone on the phone. People can actually feel your smile through the receiver. Try it!

2. Keep your answers relevant—The best way to accomplish relevance is to listen to what the interviewer is asking for. You should be certain not to cut the interviewer off before he or she finishes speaking, but you should also focus on listening by looking closely at the interviewer and making sure you don't start preparing your answer until she or he has completed asking the question. It is fine to pause for a bit before you answer. This actually makes you look more thoughtful.

    Additionally, answer the question based on what you hear, not on what you want to say. Remember, we have two ears and one mouth for a reason.

3. Be empathetic—A key trait of a physician assistant is empathy. You must show a sincere interest in others' feelings if you are going to be an effective medical provider. Empathy will help you connect with the interviewers on a "gut" level and enhance the likeability factor. At the end of each interview, they will ask you if you have any questions for them. Ask about the three most important expectations for being a PA student and why they are important. Show that you understand the logical and emotional implications of achieving those expectations.

4. Genuine—Be true to yourself and your values. Do not be a chameleon, agreeing with everything that the interviewers say. Use your beliefs and value system in a positive way to exude your uniqueness. Let the committee know that there is no other applicant there that day quite like you. Recall your unique selling proposition (USP) from the previous chapter, and focus on that theme throughout your interview.

MISTAKE #3: SENSE OF ENTITLEMENT

I have a name for those applicants who have a great résumé, but lack the interpersonal skills necessary to make a favorable impression at the interview. I call them "paper stars." They look phenomenal on paper—they have excellent GPAs, great GRE's, and years of medical experience—yet they lack the "people skills" necessary to win over the committee. Why? These applicants have a sense of entitlement and a false sense of security, thinking they deserve a position in next year's class because of their "hard skills." Your hard skills may get you to the dance, but it's your "soft skills" that will get you accepted to the program.

How to Avoid Having a Sense of Entitlement

Here are just a few things that you can do in order to avoid appearing to have a sense of entitlement at your interview:

1. Show some humility. Let the committee know that you remain teachable. If you know everything, you cannot learn anything.
2. Don't assume anything. Just because you may be a chiropractor or a foreign medical graduate, it doesn't mean you'll be a good PA. Stay open to suggestions and recommendations.
3. Never speak badly about your competition. The committee is interested in what you have to offer. Being judgmental will be detrimental to your interview score.
4. Never speak badly about another profession. Knocking the nursing profession especially is the kiss of death for any PA school applicant. PAs are team players who work in collaboration with many health-care professionals. Don't alienate yourself from other team members. Additionally, chances

are high that one of your interviewers is married to a nurse, was a nurse in a former life, or has a mom who is a nurse.

5. Don't push your own agenda. It is okay to be assertive, but being aggressive will turn off the interviewer. Answer the questions being asked without spinning the answer to meet your needs.

MISTAKE #4: FAILURE TO MAKE AN EMOTIONAL CONNECTION

By the time you make it to the interview, you have significantly increased your odds of being accepted. You have met all of the requirements on paper with respect to grades, test scores, and medical experience. Your goal now is to make an emotional connection with the admissions committee, in person. You need to transcend your résumé and convince your interviewer(s) to select you over other applicants.

The ability to communicate effectively is the single most important skill you will need to succeed as a PA. If you have a 4.0 GPA and eight thousand hours of medical experience, yet you speak in a monotone voice and avoid eye contact, you are not going to connect with the interviewer and you will most likely not receive a favorable score. The interview is an opportunity to showcase your skills and abilities and to make that all-important emotional connection that will enhance your chances of success.

If there is one "secret" to succeeding at the interview, it is this: *the admissions committee selects candidates on the basis of emotion and justifies its decision with the facts.* In other words, you cannot rely solely on your résumé to close the deal at the interview; you will need to be likeable, credible, and trustworthy.

How to Make an Emotional Connection

Creating an emotional impact is the key to your success as a PA school applicant. Personal impact is power! Consider these three crucial points prior to your interview:

1. If you want to make an emotional impact with the admissions committee and motivate and persuade them to select you for the next class, you must learn to master the spoken word.

2. People must believe what you say in order for you to have impact. If you don't believe this, just watch Bill O'Reilly on Fox news. Every week, he has an expert on "body language" (Tonya Reiman), and she can tell if people are lying by the subtleties in their facial expressions, eye contact, or posture.

3. Believability is determined at the subconscious level. One trick to making yourself more believable is to smile, make eye contact, and use open gestures.

The interview process can be extremely anxiety-provoking, and you may feel like you are in a fishbowl throughout the day. However, the more prepared you are to make that emotional connection with the committee, the less you will have to worry about.

Preparation can be the key to making the emotional connection as well. Here are three important points to remember:

1. Before the interview, do your homework. Do a Web search on the PA program. Try to find out as much as you can about the program—the mission of the program, the focus of the program (primary care, underserved areas, surgical), first-time pass/fail rates, faculty, etc. Additionally, do a Google search on the faculty and staff members who will be conducting your interview. The more you know about the program and the faculty, the better chance you have of making an emotional connection.

2. During the interview, look and listen. Stay aware of your interviewer's body language, especially signs of excitement (leaning forward, smiling). Pick up on it, and make a mental note, so you can include it in your thank-you letter. Also, be sure to allow the interviewer time to finish speaking before you attempt to answer a question. If you cut the interviewer off midsentence, you will be sending a strong message of invalidation. Be sure to maintain eye contact and use open gestures. Answer the question, but do not ramble.

3. After the interview, send a thank-you note. Write down the names of everyone with whom you interviewed. Send them all a handwritten note to thank them and to cover any points that you didn't address during the interview. If you made an emotional connection with any of the interviewers, allude to it in the note to reinforce that connection. Keep the note brief and to the point.

MISTAKE #5: INAPPROPRIATE DRESS/ACCESSORIES

Although some of you may not think it is fair, the reality is that well-kempt people receive special attention from teachers, the legal system, and employers. Attractive people earn more. In fact, researchers found that attractive, put-together people tend to earn 5 percent more. Well-groomed, put-together people are viewed as honest and helpful, while unattractive people are viewed as rude and unfair.

You only get two seconds to make a first impression on your interviewer, and if you blow it, it can take thirty minutes to recover. Given that most interviews only last twenty minutes, you cannot afford to take any chances.

What to Wear

Here are ten tips to help you enhance your visual message on the day of your interview:

1. Formal versus casual—It is better to err on being too formal than too informal. I strongly recommend a business suit for men and women.
2. Dress conservatively. Interviewing for PA school is different than interviewing for a "creative" position. Avoid scarves, nose rings, tongue rings, streaked hair, and flashy makeup.
3. Be modest. Be sure that your clothes are tailored and pressed. Skirts should hang above the knee and should not hike up too high when you are sitting.
4. Wear a jacket. You do not have to show up for your interview wearing an Armani suit; however, a jacket is a must if you want to look polished. Also, make sure your jacket fits.
5. Suit versus separates—I always recommend that applicants wear suits. Women should generally opt for a skirt-suit versus a pantsuit. However, if you feel much more comfortable in a pantsuit, by all means, wear one.
6. Keep the colors neutral. Appropriate suit colors include navy, black, grey, brown, olive, and caramel. A subtle pinstripe is also appropriate. Stay away from bold colors.
7. Wear good shoes. Be sure that your shoes are shined and neutral. Women should keep shoe styles to closed-toed, heeled sling-backs, pumps, Mary Janes, and oxfords.
8. Limit the accessories. The interview is not a fashion show. Avoid flashy jewelry, chunky necklaces, and bracelets. Remember, you want the interviewer to focus on you, not your "Jimmy Choos."

9. Well-groomed hair—Be sure that your hair is clean and secured in place. Nothing is more distracting than watching someone constantly pull strands of hair from her face.

10. Well-manicured hands/nails—Only 10 percent of your skin will be visible at the interview. Be sure to trim and clean your fingernails. Be sure that your manicure is fresh, and use conservative colors.

Although it is okay to bring a briefcase or portfolio, I recommend that you not bring it with you into the interview room. It could be distracting, and you may be tempted to fidget with it.

Finally, you can always check with the PA program to find out about the recommended attire. In fact, many programs publish this information on their Web sites. When in doubt, dress up!

Traditional Questions

3

Before we get into the interview questions and answers, I would like to touch on a key factor in establishing credibility and inspiring enthusiasm and trust at the interview.

Researchers generally agree that the spoken word is made up of three components: the verbal, the vocal, and the visual. Most applicants focus on the verbal component, but it's the visual component that actually has the most impact. In the visual message, it's the emotion and expression of your body and face as you speak that carries the most weight.

The eye is the only sensory organ that contains brain cells. Research shows that it's the visual image that makes the greatest impact in communication.

The degree of consistency or inconsistency among the verbal, vocal, and visual components of your message determines its believability. The more these three factors harmonize at the interview, the more believable you will be as a candidate. If you send mixed signals, your message may not reach the emotional center of the interviewer's brain, and you won't make that critical emotional connection.

The three components of the spoken message are quantified as follows:

- Verbal = 7 percent
- Voice = 38 percent
- Visual = 55 percent

The take-home message is that you can significantly increase or decrease your chances of scoring high at the interview by simply enhancing the visual component of your message: dress appropriately, make good eye contact, smile, avoid facial tics and inappropriate mannerisms, and maintain good posture at all times.

TRADITIONAL QUESTIONS

Traditional questions are "traditionally" the most commonly asked questions at a PA school interview. They are also the easiest to prepare for since almost every PA program asks similar questions in this format.

THE PURPOSE OF TRADITIONAL PA SCHOOL INTERVIEW QUESTIONS

Traditional interview questions allow the interviewer to get a feel for your:

- Knowledge of the PA profession
- Reasons for choosing the PA profession
- Personality
- Seriousness as an applicant (Are you just "testing the water"? Or are you a serious candidate?)
- Communication skills
- Interpersonal skills
- "Fitness" for the program

By knowing the most commonly asked questions ahead of time, you will be more confident and less anxious.

Let's start first with the most important question you'll be asked: "Why do you want to become a physician assistant?"

You can count on being asked this question at the interview. I can't tell you how many applicants I have seen who looked like a deer caught in the headlights when I asked this basic question. I wondered, *How can anyone go into a PA school interview and be surprised by this question?*

I recommend that you prepare your answer to this question and be able to recite that answer as easily as you can recite your date of birth! Be sure not to give overused, generalized answers that don't answer the question.

Also, keep in mind that the question is why do you want to become a physician assistant? It is *not* why do you want to work in health-care? Your answer should be relevant and specific to becoming a physician assistant.

There is a reason why I stress this point. Many PA school applicants will start answering the question as follows: "I've always been fascinated by medicine…" or

"Working in health care is very rewarding..." or "I love helping people..." These answers are not relevant to becoming a physician assistant.

Another thing *not* to do is recite the American Academy of Physician Assistants (AAPA) definition of a PA: "PAs are health-care professionals licensed to practice medicine..." Remember that your audience (interviewers) is a group of PAs, and they know the definition of a PA. Additionally, citing the AAPA definition of a PA does not answer the question!

To help you formulate your personal answer to this question, I recommend that you get out a piece of paper and answer the following questions:

1. Why don't I want to become a physician?
2. Why don't I want to become a nurse?
3. Why don't I want to become a nurse practitioner?
4. Why don't I want to become a firefighter? They "help" people.

By writing down your answers to these questions, you will find it much easier to narrow down your reasons for wanting to become a PA.

SAMPLE QUESTIONS

In order to help you learn how to answer interview questions effectively, I'll be giving you a round of sample questions with possible answers in the next part of this chapter. Select which answer you believe to be the best before looking at the next page. Turn the page to see if you selected the best answer and then read my explanation for why the answer may or may not be best. After you are finished with all the questions in the chapter, tally the number of correct answers and divide them by the number of total questions to see the percentage of questions you answered correctly.

In the next chapters, you will be able to do the same thing with the other types of questions. You can tally your percentages from these chapters and have a good feel for how well prepared you are for the majority of questions you'll be asked.

TRADITIONAL QUESTIONS AND ANSWERS

1. "So, why do you want to become a PA?"

Select the strongest answer.

A.) I have always been fascinated by medicine. I really enjoy helping people, and I think I'm extremely good at it. I'm a quick learner, a good communicator, and I have the ability to place patients at ease. I am not afraid of hard work or going the extra mile to get things done. I have a 3.78 science GPA, and I don't feel that I would have any problem with the didactic portion of the program. I would also be a good classmate.

B.) I believe that the PA profession is the wave of the future. The Bureau of Labor Statistics projects 39 percent job growth through 2018. The demand for good health-care providers is certainly there, and I think I can contribute to the increasing demand for health-care services. I also like the fact that I can practice medicine without having to spend the ten or more years it takes to become a physician. Additionally, I will only accumulate a fraction of the debt that physicians accumulate during the course of training.

C.) Although I enjoy my role as a registered nurse, I feel that I am ready to move on in my career. I get frustrated at times when my ability to help my patients is limited by my capacity as a nurse. I would like to learn more about the practice of medicine and be able to work in a newly enhanced position as a medical provider. At my age, it would not be practical to consider medical school because of the time and costs involved. As a PA, I can fulfill my desire to practice medicine and complete a program in two years with considerably less debt. I would also welcome the dependent nature of the profession, as I currently work in collaboration with many medical providers in all specialty areas now.

The Strongest Answer

(C) This is the strongest answer. The best way to persuade the interviewers that you are the best person for the job is to present yourself as being as close a match to the requirements as possible. Let them know that you are a good match by telling them about your skills, particularly in the specific areas required. If you have something additional to bring to the job, that will make a difference; it may be the deciding factor in whether you get accepted. Quoting colleagues or bosses helps prove your point without you having to say it explicitly.

The Mediocre Answer

(B) This is not as strong as answer (C), but it has the right tone. Consider stating one or two strong points that you have outside the job description—an "added value." This answer also shows strong confidence in yourself and your ability to do the job.

The Weakest Answer

(A) This answer is the weakest answer because it has a desperate tone. It's also very cliché ("I have always been fascinated by medicine."). It's a difficult sell when you do not have the requirements for the job. This answer does demonstrate an eager attitude and a proven ability to learn quickly, which is the right approach to take when you are lacking skills.

Limited in role as MHT

Inkling to be in healthcare

In 2 years, I can assume more responsibility

Work in a flexible position that

serves big role in healthcare

skillset appropriate for PA

2. "Tell us something about yourself."

Select the strongest answer.

A.) I was born in New England and grew up on a dairy farm. My mother was an x-ray technician, and my father ran the farm. I have three brothers and two sisters. I attended public schools and joined the navy at age seventeen. I was a navy corpsman attached to the 2nd Marine Division at Camp Lejeune, North Carolina. After an honorable discharge from the navy, I attended Southern Connecticut State University and graduated with a degree in biochemistry. I then went back into the military and joined the air force as an officer. I currently work as an EMT.

B.) I have four years' experience as a navy corpsman and three years' experience as an air force officer. As a navy corpsman, I often worked autonomously under imperfect conditions and mostly without direct physician supervision. As a junior air force officer, I was regularly tasked with many projects in which I was responsible for up to one hundred subordinates and needed to lead by example. From both experiences, I learned to work under stress, I learned to exhibit excellent communication and interpersonal skills, and I learned how to be a team player and a team leader.

C.) Sure, would you like me to focus on my personal life or my professional life?

The Best Answer

(B) This is the strongest answer because it presents a good summary of what you have to offer. The interviewer knows your total years of experience, the types of places where you have worked, and what you consider your strengths relative to a job. The answer also provides a good blend of knowledge-based skills, transferable skills, and some personality traits. You are striving to give the interviewer a good snapshot of yourself.

The Mediocre Answer

(A) This answer is okay, but it is not as strong as answer (B). This is basically a "summation of your résumé" type answer. "I was born, attended the military, attended college, and worked at…" It would benefit from more detail and specifics, such as types of companies you worked for or some of your strengths and personal characteristics. The ideal answer contains a well-rounded, current picture of you.

The Weakest Answer

(C) This is a very common reply to this question, but it is a weak answer. It does not show any preparation or planning in regard to figuring out what the committee would be interested in knowing about you. Your reply to this question is your opportunity to lead the interview and start out by focusing on what you want the interviewer to know about you and your qualifications for becoming a PA school student.

3. "Why do you want to attend our program?"

Select the strongest answer.

A.) I did some research and selected the schools that most interested me, and yours is at the top of my list. I researched PA programs based on interviews with current students, first-time pass/fail rates on the NCCPA boards, longevity of the program, and clinical rotation sites. I feel that your program meets my criteria for what I am looking for in a strong program. I know that I would be a good fit at this school and that I have a lot to contribute.

B.) I found your school in the PA programs directory. This school is a perfect fit for my educational background and medical experience. I see this program as one that will challenge me. I want to attend a program with a reputation like yours and where I can make a contribution to the student population. I know that I would be a good "fit" here.

C.) When I saw your listing in the PA programs directory, I knew I wanted to attend PA school here. My uncle is an alumnus of this school, and I would really like to be able to say I graduated from here too. It's important to me that a PA program has a good reputation and a good educational program. I see this school as a great opportunity for me to become a PA and graduate from a top-notch program.

The Best Answer

(A) This is the strongest answer because it demonstrates planning and control on your part, not just an attitude of "there was an opportunity so I thought I would apply." You demonstrate that you have given some thought to what you want and how to go about getting it. You selected this program by doing research and taking the time to speak with some current students. This answer shows confidence in your skills and ability to fit into this program. You need to be aware of the fact that you may be walking a thin line here. You need to project confidence, while not being overconfident.

The Mediocre Answer

(C) This is a very mediocre answer. It emphasizes "you" and what you can get from the opportunity. While being a fan of the school is good from a PR standpoint, the answer would be stronger if you mentioned some specifics about the program and why you would be a good fit for this school. Simply being a fan of the school does not get you any extra points in the interview process. A little flattery goes a long way, but make sure you are looking at the program for the right reasons.

The Weakest Answer

(B) This is a selfish answer. The emphasis is on "what's in it for me?" The bottom line of the interview process is "What can you contribute to this class?" not "What can our program do for you?"

4. "What are your goals as a PA?"

Select the strongest answer.

A.) My goal is to graduate from a good PA program and eventually work as a senior PA. I would like to lead a team of PAs in a surgical arena. I see myself heading up a burn team in a cutting-edge hospital one day.

B.) I want to first work in a multispecialty group that believes in cross-training. I think this is the best way to achieve a strong foundation in medicine. I would then like to consider a postgraduate training program where I can specialize and become a leader in my chosen field.

C.) I've always believed in short-, medium-, and long-term goals. Right now, I'd like to attend a strong PA program, graduate, and be able to pass my boards. I then would like to work on a team and gain as much generalized knowledge of medicine as possible. Long-term goals will depend on my experiences along the way. I will look for opportunities that will continue to be challenging and where I can make a significant contribution in the health-care profession.

The Best Answer

(C) This is the strongest answer among the three choices. Since this is an open-ended question, there is no right or wrong way to answer it. This answer is best because it shows the candidate is open to opportunities that allow room for growth but doesn't lock the speaker into goals that may be unrealistic or are too rigid or specific.

The Mediocre Answer

(B) This answer starts out well, but then gets a little too specific. It also does not take into account any other possibilities that may open up as a result of multispecialty training.

The Weakest Answer

(A) This answer is a bit ambitious for someone just entering the field. It is very narrow-minded and would probably be a turnoff to the interviewer.

5. "What do you consider your strengths?"

Select the strongest answer.

A.) My biggest strength is that I am a people person. I love helping people and providing comfort. My patients are very important to me, and I let them know it. I frequently receive compliments from my patients and my supervisors alike.

B.) My strengths are a combination of my interpersonal skills and my ability to communicate with staff and patients alike. I am a team player and consider myself a great listener. I think what separates me from the competition, though, is my ability to put my patients and their families at ease. I have the ability to break down complex medical data into simple, yet concise terminology. I was voted "employee of the year" the last two years as a direct result of patient and employee feedback.

C.) I am a great communicator. Whether working with my health-care team or dealing with patients, I have a cooperative style that contributes to the mission or task at hand. As a result, I was voted "employee of the year" the last two years in a row.

The Best Answer

(B) This is the strongest answer because it paints a broader picture of what you bring to the profession—that is, not only what is required (technical skills) but also the added value of being able to work directly with patients as well as a strong ability to communicate technical information in simple terms. In this competitive PA profession, it will be necessary for you to think of your strengths beyond meeting qualifications. What else can you offer that other applicants cannot? The more skills you include in your answer, the more information the interviewer will have to judge whether you have what it takes to do the job—and beyond.

The Mediocre Answer

(C) This answer is not as strong an answer as (B). It is good in that it lets the interviewer know that you have a strong ability to work with patients and co-workers alike. This answer would be stronger if you blended in some of the skills that come from your experience or knowledge, such as your medical or technical knowledge.

The Weakest Answer

(A) This is a very general answer that could be used for any position. "I am a people person" and "I love helping people" are overused phrases. Why don't you want to become a physician? Physicians are "people persons" and "love helping people" too.

6. "What is your greatest weakness?"

Select the strongest answer.

A.) I believe that "we bring about what we think about," so I don't dwell on weaknesses. However, I would have to say that being impatient in dealing with those who don't "catch on" as quickly as I do is one of my weak points. I've learned to enlist the cooperation of my co-workers and to demonstrate quicker ways to get the job done. Leading by example is a much more effective way of dealing with impatience than holding in my frustrations.

B.) I am a person who likes to get the job done correctly the first time. I become frustrated when other people's work affects my ability to do my job correctly. I've been working on trying to be more understanding and finding out what the problem is before I pass judgment.

C.) My weakness is working too hard to get the job done. Because of the workload, I have to work many evenings so that projects meet deadlines. I'm trying to work smarter and not harder.

The Best Answer

(A) This answer comes across as being very sincere and honest. Some forethought was put into the answer. It also shows an awareness of your need to improve and what action steps you need to take to work through the issue.

The Mediocre Answer

(B) This is not a bad answer. However, the interviewer could become concerned that you are a bit of a perfectionist, and that could cause a problem. Avoid mentioning personality traits that would be difficult to change. In answering this question it is best to demonstrate something you are working on to improve your weakness: "I'm working on it."

The Weakest Answer

(C) This is a very trite answer and should be avoided. "Working too hard" is overused and meaningless. Additionally, an interviewer might be concerned about whether you are working hard because of the workload or because of poor work habits.

7. "How would you describe your personality?"

Select the strongest answer.

A.) I have high energy, and I am a hard worker. I learn very quickly and adapt well. I am very responsible about deadlines. I have the ability to get along well with people. I have a very upbeat attitude that helps keep my department's morale up. I have the ability to get along well with everyone.

B.) I'm a high-energy person who is motivated by new challenges and problems. I can hit the ground running and come up to speed faster than anyone I know. I have a proven record of success and a strong work ethic. My attitude about work is to be a team player and do whatever it takes to get the job done. I strive to help my co-workers and encourage cooperation too.

C.) I'm a problem-solver who is a whiz at analyzing data and transforming it into useful information. My strength is my ability to convert complex details into simple, understandable language. I am usually labeled the problem-solver of the group.

The Best Answer

(B) This is the strongest answer because of the energy it demonstrates. This answer describes your personality in a unique manner—not just a hard worker with a good attitude but an adaptable person with a "whatever it takes to get the job done" attitude. This is followed by an endorsement from your fellow workers of your ability to be a "team player."

The Mediocre Answer

(A) There is nothing in this answer that makes you unique. If you compare the words in answer (B) with those in answer (A), you will notice that they basically say the same thing. The difference is the added "zip." The terms used in this answer are clichéd. A high percentage of people would answer with "hard worker." If you do say you are a hard worker, it would be a stronger answer if you add that you work above and beyond what is called for. "I often work ten-hour days." Overall, this answer needs some punch.

The Weakest Answer

(C) This answer refers more to skills than your personality. It has a strong focus on analytical problem solving but is one-dimensional. By adding some personality traits that are more transferable, such as communication skills, you would give a better, more well-rounded picture of yourself.

8. "What experience do you have that qualifies you to join our program?"

Select the strongest answer.

A.) My experience is a good match with the qualifications needed to join the upcoming class. I meet all of the prerequisites for this program and then some. I think I can bring added value to this program through my understanding and knowledge of medicine, which I gained via my background as an inner-city EMT. My understanding of medical terminology and my experience working under conditions of urgency and stress would be a tremendous asset to my classmates with less hands-on training.

B.) I know I am well qualified to join your upcoming class. I have the background and necessary experience to succeed here. I want to attend this school, and I feel that this program would be a challenge and an opportunity for me. I am a person who likes to be challenged and also continue to grow and learn new skills. I am a good problem-solver. I like working on a team and contributing to solutions.

C.) With six years of experience working as an EMT, I have the necessary medical experience to qualify as a strong applicant. My strength is my leadership and communication skills. I have supervised and trained new technicians on a 24/7 schedule. I am also able to give brief, yet concise information to ER personnel when bringing in a sick or injured patient. If you were to ask my staff members about me, they would tell you that I am extremely dependable and loyal. I am very adaptable and have worked several seventy-hour workweeks during periods of need.

The Best Answer

(C) This is the strongest answer. The answer gives a broad picture of you and how your skills would fill the interviewer's needs. It gives examples of strengths in the area of medical experience, leadership, and communication (which are considered transferable skills), and your willingness to do "whatever it takes to get the job done." The "third-party endorsement" from people who have worked with you is very helpful. Speaking through others' comments is a strong technique to use when you are answering questions.

The Mediocre Answer

(A) This answer has its strong points, but it does not present an overall picture like answer (C) does. Any time you can speak of bringing "added value" to a program, whether through medical terminology, people skills, or the ability to do something that most applicants cannot, you should sell it as a strong point. Depending on how important your value is to the program, this could make the difference in your being the chosen candidate.

The Weakest Answer

(B) This answer focuses too much on what the program can do for you. The emphasis is best placed on what you can offer the program. This answer would be stronger if it gave specific information about the years of experience and types of problems you solved.

9. "What do you know about this program?"

Select the strongest answer.

A.) I've done research on this program and checked out the mission and the focus of the program. I am very familiar with your didactic schedule and your clinical rotation sites. I even shadowed a few of your graduate PAs, and I have spoken to a few of your current students. I know that you have well-established rotation sites and a high 90th percentile first-time pass rate on the national boards. I know this is a program I would be very interested in attending.

B.) My interest in your program began in college when a graduate member of this school gave a lecture on the PA profession. I have researched the program online, too. I know that your program ranks in the top fifteen PA schools in the nation. I have targeted this school as one that I would like to attend.

C.) When I found your school in the PA programs directory, I wasn't really familiar with your program. I began asking a few PAs I know about this program and received excellent feedback. I have heard this program has a good standing in the community and the graduates are well respected.

The Best Answer

(A) This is the strongest answer because of the skills demonstrated—not only researching the program but digging deeper for information about the mission, the focus, and rotation sites. This answer provides information and knowledge beyond what was on the Web site.

The Mediocre Answer

(B) This is not a bad answer. There is enthusiasm for the program and a history and research. The answer lacks information on what is happening in the program, the competition, and the program's pass/fail rate on the boards. All that information could be found by searching online or in the PA programs directory.

The Weakest Answer

(C) This is the weakest answer because it does not provide any facts to talk about. Unfortunately, it's not unusual for candidates to lack information about the program. At the very least, a visit to the Web site is essential. Relying on the "word" from PAs is not doing research. This answer also focuses on "the benefits" of attending a program not on the program itself.

10. "What do you value most in a classmate or co-worker?"

Select the strongest answer.

A.) I've worked with many people, and the ones who are of the most value to me are those who are dependable. One of my pet peeves is to hand off a project to someone and find out it was never accomplished. I don't understand how some people can keep their jobs when they can't be depended upon to complete the job.

B.) I really value teammates who are supportive and willing to go the extra mile to accomplish the task at hand. Once while I was working as an ER technician, we were really shorthanded on the busiest night of the year. Even though many of us had completed our shifts, we stayed late to help the rest of the physicians, nurses, and fellow technicians cope with the heavy surge of patients. We stayed until things settled down, and everyone appreciated our cooperation and dedication.

C.) I value communication skills in any work I do, but especially when I'm working with a team. I think it is necessary for all members of the team to be able to express themselves in a clear manner and be able to listen and follow directions. When communication breaks down, there is no team. Language skills are the most important part of any team effort.

The Best Answer

(B) This is the strongest answer because it gives a clear example that backs up your opinion. The answer is secondary to the message it conveys. Teamwork means getting along and working together.

The Mediocre Answer

(A) This answer could be viewed as complaining or negative. Being dependable is an important trait, but the answer would be stronger if it were phrased in a more positive manner. "I value dependability from teammates because it means the work gets completed and everyone benefits."

The Weakest Answer

(C) This answer takes on a life of its own and goes down a different path. The answer deals more with effective communication than with "the value of a teammate." The answer is not a wrong answer—communication skills are very desirable. It just doesn't relate to the question being asked.

11. "How have you stayed current and informed about the PA profession?"

Select the strongest answer.

A.) I do all of the standard things. I read the *Journal of the American Academy of Physician Assistants* (*JAAPA*); I attend some of the state chapter meetings of the AAPA—in my state, it's ConnAPA. I belong to forums on the Web for PA school students and applicants. I also shadow PAs and learn firsthand the current challenges of the PA profession. In general, I've become a student of the profession, and I am very passionate and excited about the opportunity to become a PA.

B.) I visit the AAPA Web site and some PA forums on the Web. I don't get any specific journals, but I check the newspapers for articles relative to health care and the PA profession specifically. I feel that I am more informed than the average person.

C.) I don't have a lot of free time after working and going to school at night. My busy life does not allow for much more than an occasional Web search and watching the news. I occasionally read some medical journals that I come across.

The Best Answer

(A) This answer has a very natural and relaxed tone to it, yet it covers every possible base and states that you are a person who is "out there" and informed. By being involved in groups and organizations, you are also widening your network, which is the number-one way to get accepted. Of course, in your interview, you'd give the specific names of newsletters and organizations.

The Mediocre Answer

(B) This answer is not a bad one; it just limits your information by the sources you use to stay informed. You are correct that you are probably more informed than the average person, but you are competing to be above-average in the interview process. Often a program is seeking someone who is connected to the industry, and admissions committees look at the groups to which you belong.

The Weakest Answer

(C) Although this might be a "real" answer, this is not the strongest position to be in as an informed person. Regardless of your schedule, staying informed about the latest trends and issues is crucial for job success.

12. "If I asked your co-workers or fellow students to say three positive things about you, what would they say?"

Select the strongest answer.

A.) They would most likely say that I am very knowledgeable about my job and willing to share my knowledge with them whenever they need help. Second, they would tell you that I have great organizational skills; I plan ahead and meet schedules. The third thing they would tell you is that I know when to laugh. I've learned through experience that you can't take situations too seriously.

B.) I'm not really sure what they would say. We all work together but don't have much social interaction. I think that they would tell you that I am a hard worker, because I am. I think they would tell you I am a thoughtful person—at least I try to be. And I think they would say I am a team player. I always try to help others.

C.) That's not an easy question. I think they think I am responsible. I'm always cooperative. I don't gossip or get involved in company politics. On the negative side, some of them think I'm aloof because I don't get involved in the gossip. But I think it is best to keep work and social life separate.

The Strongest Answer

(A) This is the strongest answer not only because of the examples but because the skills named are a mixture of skills. You gave an example of your work knowledge; your organizational skills, which can be applied in any profession; and your personal traits, which make you a likeable person. It's best when you can give a mixture of skills and traits. That is what makes you unique.

The Mediocre Answer

(B) This answer would be stronger if you gave some reasons for the answers, such as, "They would tell you I am a very thoughtful person. I always remember everyone's birthday and send a card or a little gift." When you give an example with the statement, it makes more of an impact. Also, avoid the phrase "I think." It makes you appear less confident.

The Weakest Answer

(C) This answer is weak because it does not have a positive viewpoint and turns negative at the end. Never volunteer a negative thought about yourself unless you are asked for a weakness. This answer does not give the impression that you are much of a team player.

13. "If it comes down to you and one other applicant, why should we select you?"

Select the strongest answer.

A.) I can be a great PA; I know I can. Because I am a quick learner, I have the ability to pick up things faster than most people can. I am currently taking classes in medical terminology and anatomy and physiology to prepare myself and learn the things I don't know. I will be a great student and be able to contribute to the class immediately. I am looking for an opportunity to show how committed I am to being a PA.

B.) My strong sense of compassion and communication skills is what I can bring to this program. I have an ability to connect with people and make them feel at ease. My current patients in Dr. Brown's office often bring me small gifts to show their appreciation for my caring for them. When I learned about this school, I knew it was the school for me.

C.) If you compare my qualifications with your requirements, you will see that I am almost a perfect match for your program. I have the required GPA and test scores. I have more than enough quality hours of hands-on medical experience. I have a full understanding of the PA role. I've shadowed five of your graduate students, and I understand the philosophy and focus of your program. If you were to ask those five PAs to say something about me, they would tell you, "She has a strong desire to become a PA, and she would be a great fit for this program."

The Strongest Answer

(C) This is the strongest answer because it focuses on the requirements and pre-requisites of the program, including GPA and medical experience. It also tells the interviewer what you have specifically done to improve your chances of acceptance. This answer shows motivation, maturity, and enthusiasm.

The Mediocre Answer

(A) This answer is okay, but not as strong as (C). It does mention the fact that you would be able to "contribute to the class," which is a trait programs look for in applicants. However, the answer should focus more on your qualifications and background to demonstrate the fact that you can complete a rigorous program of study.

The Weakest Answer

(B) This is the weakest answer because it is too vague and does not get specific enough about your qualifications. It's important to be a compassionate person, but you have to explain why the interviewer should select you over another applicant. This response does not get the job done!

14. "Do you have any questions?"

Select the strongest answer.

A.) I would like to know about the scholarships you offer and how the program decides who will receive one. I would also like to know more about paid work opportunities in the area.

B.) You and the rest of the committee have been very thorough about the program expectations. I don't have any further questions at this time. I'm sure I may have more questions once I start the program.

C.) One thing that has been talked about during the interview is the philosophy of the program. Can you explain to me more about that and how it came about?

The Strongest Answer

(C) This is the strongest answer because it shows that you have been listening and are aware that one of the first things you need to understand is the "philosophy" of the program. The bottom line of the interview is to see if you're a good fit for the program. If you understand the philosophy and focus of the program, you can see if you're a good match for the program and if the program is a good match for you. This leads the interviewer to believe that you are interviewing the school as well as the school interviewing you.

The Mediocre Answer

(A) Depending on where you are in the interview process, this answer could be appropriate. This would be a good question to ask in a first interview before any interest is shown. This question focuses on what you will get out of attending the school. You will need the information eventually; just wait until the appropriate time to bring it up, such as after you've been offered a place in the upcoming class.

The Weakest Answer

(B) This is the most common reply used by applicants—"No, I don't have any questions"—and it is the wrong answer. It is very important that you ask questions to show your interest and let the interviewer know you have been listening.

15. "If I remember one thing about you, what should that be?"

Select the strongest answer.

A.) I have an unusual hobby that you might remember me mentioning. I am an off-Broadway actress, and I can tie a cherry stem into a knot with my tongue. I have made a lot of money taking bets on that one!

B.) I can be remembered for my passion. Anything I set my mind to I can bring about through persistence and drive. I can focus on a task and see it through to the end.

C.) I have two skills that are distinctly different but that define my personality. I am a very good classical guitar player and an excellent mechanic; I'm known for having strong, steady hands.

The Strongest Answer

(C) This is the strongest answer, especially if your goal is to work in surgery where "good hands" are a requirement. Obviously, you will not necessarily be able to relate your hobbies to your job, but you can see how this would make the interviewer remember you after you finish the interview. The idea is to find something that sets you apart from everyone else. And if the interviewer happens to play guitar or be a good mechanic, you've hit a home run!

The Mediocre Answer

(B) This answer is okay, but not terribly interesting or memorable. In fact, it's rather cliché. There is a risk-benefit to sticking out your neck to use an answer like (C) above, but it could mean the difference between acceptance and rejection.

The Weakest Answer

(A) This is the weakest answer because it is way over the edge. The part about being an off-Broadway actress is interesting, but the "cherry stem" trick is totally inappropriate—memorable, but inappropriate.

16. "Have you applied to any other programs?"

Select the strongest answer.

A.) No, I haven't. I want to attend this program, and I will do what it takes to get accepted.

B.) Yes, I have. I have applied to thirteen schools. I really want to become a PA, and I want to maximize my chances for acceptance. I know that competition is fierce, and I want to get into a program this year. I feel that my best chance is not by putting all of my eggs in one basket.

C.) Yes, I have applied to Duke, Emory, Yale, and George Washington. I feel that these are the original programs with a strong history of educating the best PAs. The pass/fail rates are exceptional, and I can feel confident that I will be able to pass my boards after graduation. Additionally, I understand that competition for each program is keen, and I would like to maximize my chances for acceptance into a program that will provide an optimal learning experience.

The Strongest Answer

(C) This is the strongest answer because it focuses on a theme when choosing programs: "strong history of educating the best PAs." It also discusses the pass/fail rates, which are important to an applicant, who has to pass the boards. Finally, the applicant has applied to five programs, which seems to be the perfect number. It does not leave you appearing to be desperate.

The Mediocre Answer

(B) This answer is okay, but not as strong as (C). Although the applicant is certainly enthusiastic, thirteen programs are way too many; the applicant appears to be grabbing at straws without regard for the quality of the program. She just wants in to any program.

The Weakest Answer

(A) This is the weakest answer because the applicant does not seem to have a sense of urgency. Applying to only one program leaves the impression that this candidate may not be too serious about becoming a PA and may be just "testing the waters." On the other hand, some applicants have families and cannot afford to move out of state.

17. "What is a 'dependent' practitioner?"

Select the strongest answer.

A.) A dependent practitioner must work directly with a supervisor and always be at the same physical location.

B.) PAs are dependent practitioners. They are required to work with physician supervision. Although the PA must declare a supervising physician and be registered in the state of employment, he or she also may work autonomously.

C.) I guess I'm not sure what you mean by "dependent practitioner." Can you give me a little more information?

The Strongest Answer

(B) This is the strongest answer because it actually answers the question but also provides additional information into what a dependent practitioner is. It shows the interviewer that the candidate is knowledgeable about the field.

The Mediocre Answer

(A) This answer is okay, but not as strong as (B). Although the applicant is answering the question, this answer does not provide as much detailed knowledge of the role as does response B.

The Weakest Answer

(C) Even though you are being honest with this response because you really don't know, this is obviously a poor response because you should know. Make sure that you prepare enough and understand enough about the field before you get to the interview stage so that you can avoid problems like this.

18. "Why do you want to change careers?"

Select the strongest answer.

    A.) I am not making enough money in my current profession, and I would like to earn more money. I've been told you can make a lot of money being a PA.

    B.) As I have matured and experienced more, I've learned that I am very interested in health care. I interviewed individuals in several health-care fields—physicians, nurses, nurse practitioners, and PAs—and found that I am most drawn to the PA profession for many reasons. First, I like the collaborative aspect of being a PA and working in a health-care team. Yet I also like the autonomy that the PA profession would provide me. I am fascinated by the number of specialties available to PAs. Finally, I have a good deal of respect for the profession and was very impressed with the PAs I spoke with about their jobs.

    C.) I'm very interested in helping people and doing good work. I'd like to work in some type of health-care context/setting, and I thought this might be fun.

The Best Answer

(B) This is the best answer because it shows that you have researched options and selected the profession because of what it can provide you. You seem to be sincerely interested in a being a PA over other health-care careers.

The Mediocre Answer

(C) While this answer does communicate to the interviewer that you are interested in helping others, it suggests that you have no particular passion for being a PA. It also suggests that you haven't done much research into the profession. You also naively state that it might be "fun." While there may be fun elements to being a PA, it is a challenging job filled with much intensity and can be stressful at times.

The Weakest Answer

(A) This is the weakest answer because it shows that your top priority is making money. While making money is the main reason most of us work, one can make money in other professions—so why the PA profession? It also suggests that you haven't done much research into PA salaries because you say you have "been told that" PAs make a lot of money.

19. "Explain your undergraduate grades."

Select the strongest answer.

A.) I am not particularly proud of my first two years in school and don't believe that the grades from those years are at all representative of my ability to perform or of my motivation. In my first two years of school, I lacked direction and struggled to find a reason for being in class. I also worked nearly full-time, and that did impact my grades. As you can see by my transcript, my grades improved significantly once I found out what I was interested in and declared a major.

As a more mature person now, I know how to motivate myself and find the passion in most things, but as an eighteen-year-old, I lacked that skill.

B.) I was not very motivated in my first two years of college. I wasn't prepared to be on my own and didn't have good study habits. I made up for those grades in my second two years, however.

C.) I did a lot of partying as an undergraduate. I'm not proud of it, but I would be a much better student now.

The Best Answer

(A) This is the best answer because it is honest yet also explains the poor grades. The best part about the answer is that it addresses how you have changed and why this wouldn't happen to you in PA school even if you found yourself in a class that wasn't as interesting to you as you might like.

The Mediocre Answer

(B) While this answer give the interviewers some important information about why your grades suffered in the first two years, it does not give them enough to reassure them that you will continue to have good grades in PA school. You need to be able to communicate specifically how your study skills have improved and why you will continue to be motivated in PA school.

The Weakest Answer

(C) This is the weakest answer because it does little to reassure the interviewers that you will perform well in PA school. With such a brief response, they are unlikely to take a risk with someone who has not communicated to them why he is different now or how he might be different in PA school.

20. "If you had a patient with a language barrier, how would you assist that patient?"

Select the strongest answer.

A.) I would try to find someone who spoke the language to translate for me.

B.) I would muddle through as best I could. I would probably draw pictures and try to use sign language or gestures to communicate to him or her what I was doing or wishing to do.

C.) There are many things to consider when dealing with someone who has a language barrier. In addition to the language issue, the person also comes from a different culture and that culture might have different understandings and values related to health and health care.

Preparation is key. I make every effort to learn about different cultures so if I am ever in this situation, I will have a basis for understanding.

But in this situation, I would try to find a translator. Many hospitals have translators on staff. I might also try to work with family members who speak English and hope that they can assist. I would watch nonverbal communication closely and make sure that I don't upset the patient. I would try to find ways to reassure him or her (e.g., calming facial expressions, smiles, etc.). I might draw pictures and diagrams, but I would need to be sure that the patient understands my drawings.

The Best Answer

(C) This is the best answer because it includes many different considerations related to this issue. This answer shows the interviewer that you are open to learning about other cultures, are aware that this most likely will happen to you as you practice, and are prepared to be creative.

The Mediocre Answers

(A/B) While trying to find someone to translate for you and also trying to find other ways to communicate are good ideas, they are only the start of what you should do. It is far too easy to miscommunicate through gestures and drawings. Likewise, using only a translator disconnects you from the patient. You need to establish a relationship with the patient outside of the formal spoken languages you both use.

21. "What makes you mad?"

Select the strongest answer.

A.) I really don't get mad that often, but injustice is my biggest button. If I think that things are unfair, I usually get angry about that. In that situation, I assess whether or not I can make a difference, and if I can, I try to facilitate change. If I can't, I try to accept the situation and reframe it or use it as an opportunity to learn a lesson about how I will not do things or treat others.

B.) My dad was a hothead, and he used to fly off the handle at us when we were kids. My mom was afraid of him. So, as I got older, I learned to control my anger. So I generally don't show that I am mad when I am. I usually just keep it inside and control it and then blow off steam in other ways. I like to exercise and play sports, and that is typically how I get my anger out when I am mad.

C.) I don't actually ever get mad.

The Best Answer

(A) This is the best answer because it is honest. It also explains to the interviewer how you would handle your anger. You can substitute a variety of other answers for "injustice" and still be able to respond in a similar manner. The important point here is to be honest and then respond positively about how you manage your anger.

The Mediocre Answer

(B) This answer shows the interviewers that you have thought about the issue and how you express anger. However, it gives them more information than they need. Rather than talking about your parents, you could say, "I have given that some thought because I know that it is important for a health-care professional to understand how she expresses emotion," and then elaborate on your exercise strategies.

The Weakest Answer

(C) Everyone gets angry, and claiming that you don't is a mistake because the interviewer really does want to know how you respond when you are angry. With this answer, you give the interviewer no idea of how you would handle yourself in a stressful and frustrating situation.

22. "Tell me something unique about yourself that is not already included in your application."

Select the strongest answer.

A.) I am a complete Star Trek freak. I love the shows and have a complete DVD collection of all episodes. I've even attended some Star Trek conferences.

B.) I am an avid reader. I read many different types of books—fiction and nonfiction, newspapers, journals, pretty much anything I can get my hands on. This makes me a bit of a trivia expert as well.

C.) I was diagnosed with pneumonia when I was in third grade and had to be admitted to the hospital. While I was there, I was fascinated by the nurses and equipment and decided then that I wanted to work in health care.

The Best Answer

(B) This is the best answer because it adds to your value as a candidate. If you aren't an avid reader, an answer that tells the committee that you have skills and competencies related to being a good student or PA is what you should mention in this answer.

The Mediocre Answer

(C) This answer gives the interviewers some idea of why you became interested in the health-care profession. It also tells them that you have some experience being a patient. However, it does nothing to distinguish you as a candidate as it is likely that other candidates will have similar experiences (thus, it is not really unique).

The Weakest Answer

(A) You missed a great opportunity here to make a case for why you stand out from all the other applicants. Your example, while perhaps interesting to some, does nothing to advance your case for being admitted to PA school.

23. "If you could change one thing about the PA profession, as you understand it today, what would you change?"

Select the strongest answer.

      A.) I would make it so the physicians have more respect for the PAs. I don't like being talked down to, and I suspect that physicians think they can do that to PAs like they do to nurses.

      B.) I would increase the number of colleges and universities that offer PA programs. The demand for PAs still exceeds the supply, and new health-care reform laws will create a need for even more practitioners.

      C.) I wish patients understood the PA profession better. I don't think most of them know the difference between a PA and a nurse, and they sometimes miss opportunities for help because we have different roles.

The Best Answer

(B) This is the best answer because it displays an understanding of the profession, programs, and issues related to health-care reform. You look knowledgeable and well informed with this answer.

The Mediocre Answer

(C) This answer addresses a fundamental problem with the PA profession— that patients often don't understand the role and responsibilities assumed by PAs. This answer doesn't, however, display that you have a deep understanding of the profession.

The Weakest Answer

(A) While this may be a genuine concern, this answer is weak for a few reasons. First, you are assuming that all physicians treat PAs without respect, and that is an inaccurate assumption. Second, it suggests that you already have a bias on this issue and would communicate to the interviewers that you might "see" a problem that might not actually be there. Third, you have missed an opportunity to communicate your deep knowledge and understanding of the PA profession.

24. "What do you like to do outside of school?"

Select the strongest answer.

    A.) Mainly, I like to relax and have fun with friends.

    B.) I am a very involved volunteer. I volunteer at the free clinic in my neighborhood and also at the Red Cross. I organized a blood drive through my church last year.

    C.) I have many hobbies and interests. I like to spend time with my family and friends. I am a kayaker and enjoy golfing. I also enjoy making pottery. I am a volunteer at my church as well.

The Best Answer

(C) This is the best answer because it portrays you as a well-rounded person. This question is designed to understand the "you" behind the candidate. Additionally, the balance of relationships and hobbies communicates to the interviewers that you are interested in relationships and accomplishing tasks.

The Mediocre Answer

(B) While this answer tells the interviewer that you are interested in health care and have volunteered, it is a predictable response. Unless you really do like to volunteer outside of school and that is your main hobby and source of entertainment, stick to something that is more genuine and believable or make it a part of an answer that includes the rest of what you do outside of school.

The Weakest Answer

(A) Although this might be an honest answer, it does little to advance the interviewers' knowledge about who you are as a person. If you choose to talk about friends and family, you might add details about interpersonal skills and how you value close relationships and making connections with others.

25. "Which field do you see yourself working in after graduation?"

Select the strongest answer.

A.) At this point, I'm really not sure. I know I have a passion for the PA profession, but until I take classes and get some additional experience, I'm not sure what I will be interested in.

B.) I know I want to go into family medicine, because I can work with the most diverse group of people and be on the front line of the health-care profession.

C.) At this point, I'm most interested in pediatrics or family practice. I like the idea of working in general medicine and with a varied population of patients. I know that I may change my mind though as I learn more about the field.

The Best Answer

    (C) This is the best answer because it shows that you have given thought to what interests you and why, but you still leave the door open to other options as you learn more about the field and areas of specialty.

The Mediocre Answer

    (A) This answer shows that you are open to the possibilities of different options as you proceed through the program. However, it also suggests that you've not given a lot of thought to which area of the profession interests you most.

The Weakest Answer

    (B) While your reasons are clear, this is the weakest answer because you sound rigid and not open to different options as you progress through school. You want to let others know that while you may have a current preference, you are open to considering other areas as you learn about them and have more experience as a student PA.

26. "Tell me your thoughts about health-care reform."

Select the strongest answer.

A.) As someone who is interested in health care, I have been watching with
interest all that is happening in this area. I try not to get into the politics
of it though—since patient care is my only interest.

B.) I have been an adamant supporter of Obamacare. I cannot understand
how the Republicans can object to it. We are the only developed nation
in the world that does not provide health coverage for our citizens.

C.) I personally believe that everyone in the United States should have
access to quality health care. As far as the means by which we, as a
country, bring this plan to fruition, that is a political decision versus a
personal one for me.

Adds efficiency to the healthcare system
Increase availablity of physician services

The Best Answer

(C) This is the best answer because you answer the question without taking a political position. You aren't in the interview to discuss politics (as mentioned before) and this answer explains your values without getting into the politics of how access to quality care can be achieved.

The Mediocre Answer

(A) This answer shows that you have been following the debate. While not discussing politics during the interview is a good idea, your answer gives the interviewers no idea how you see health-care reform and patient care matching up. It also looks as if you don't really know about the issues but want to pretend you do.

The Weakest Answer

(B) This answer shows that you are passionate about the issue, but it is a risky response. While some interviewers may be in complete agreement, others might not be. Also, you have missed an opportunity to talk about health care in a general sense, and if you are as passionate as you seem to be, you have many important thoughts about health care that the committee would be happy to hear.

27. "Do you think health-care reform will be positive or negative for physician assistants? Why or why not?"

Select the strongest answer.

A.) I think health-care reform will be a "positive" for physician assistants. With current plans to extend health insurance coverage to some forty-seven million people, coupled with the current primary-care physician shortage, PAs will be in more demand than ever.

B.) Yes. Saving money is a big part of health-care reform, and since PAs bill at a less expensive rate than physicians, PAs will be in greater demand. I see it as a positive for the profession.

C.) No. I don't think that health-care reform will make any difference to PAs.

Benefits the patients the main
focus for PAs.

The Best Answer

(A) This is the best answer because it presents the factual data to explain the reality of the health-care reform situation. It also shows that you have done your homework when it comes to health-care reform.

The Mediocre Answer

(B) While there may be some logic to your answer, it is mediocre because it is a simplistic response to a complex question. Undoubtedly, the PA profession will be impacted by health-care reform, and the impact may include many things beyond issues related to demand. You also miss an opportunity to communicate to the interviewers that you understand the complexity of health-care reform.

The Weakest Answer

(C) You might respond this way if you wish to avoid a discussion of politics related to health-care reform. But this answer is wrong. Health-care reform will impact all Americans and every type of health-care worker. Saying it won't is simply naive.

28. "Do you think the physician assistant profession should change its name to physician associate? Why or why not?"

Select the strongest answer.

A.) No, I don't think so. People know PAs as physician assistants, and so it would be confusing to change the name.

B.) I personally feel that PAs should be called physician associates as opposed to physician assistants. In 1965, the profession's original name was physician associate, and the name change occurred only as a result of some concerns by physicians. I believe that forty years later, the PA's role is better served by the name "physician associate," because the word "assistant" is a very generic term that can be quite misleading.

C.) I think that would be a good idea. *Assistant* sounds too low level for the work we do, and we need to have credibility with patients and other health-care providers. Maybe nurses would respect us more if we were "associates" rather than "assistants."

The Best Answer

(B) This is the best answer because it shows you have done your homework on the profession. Likewise, you make a sound argument for why the name should be changed from *assistant* to *associate*.

The Mediocre Answer

(A) This answer shows you have some understanding of the impact this might have on patients. However, it is a simplistic answer and isn't likely to "wow" the interviewers.

The Weakest Answer

(C) First, making a derogatory comment about nurses creates a major strike against you. Second, while credibility is important, this answer makes you sound like you believe that you can gain credibility through your title, rather than actions.

29. "Should all PA programs be master's-level programs?"

Select the strongest answer.

A.) Yes, definitely. A master's degree prepares one for the demands of being a PA. I know that my master's program was important for me because I had to take responsibility for my learning as well as meet deadlines. I also learned how to work in a team on group assignments.

B.) I'm not sure that a master's degree is necessary. Both the bachelor's and master's are important, but the master's may not be necessary.

C.) The trend toward master's level PA programs started many years ago. Currently, the majority of PA programs are at the master's level. It is difficult to say that *all* PA programs should be master's-level because most of the PAs who were pioneers of the profession did not have master's degrees. However, I do believe that a strong case can be made that the rigorous didactic and clinical training in PA school warrants a master's degree.

The Best Answer

(C) This is the best answer because it clearly identifies the complexity of the question noting that it would be hard to make master's degrees mandatory. However, the answer also acknowledges that the material covered in PA programs is challenging and certainly warrants a master's level rating. This tells the interviewer that you are well aware of the rigorous didactic nature of programs.

The Mediocre Answer

(A) This answer begins to address some of the skills and attributes one can attain by completing a master's degree. However, it emphasizes "you" rather than the PA profession.

The Weakest Answer

(B) This answer is vague and indecisive. You really don't answer the question by committing to one or the other, and it sounds like you are trying to avoid the answer.

30. "Do you think HMOs and PPOs are good or bad for the PA profession?"

Select the strongest answer.

A.) They can be good for the profession because they work to make medical care more cost effective. They also encourage responsible behavior by placing limits on treatment options, and that can be a good thing because some physicians are unethical and prescribe too many procedures.

B.) I believe HMOs and PPOs are good for the PA profession because PAs are cost effective and yet rank highly in terms of patient satisfaction.

C.) No, I don't think it is a good thing. It creates a lot of paperwork for PAs, and we are already too busy to deal with paperwork.

health → Health maintenance organization

Preferred provider organization

prevent you but ?
allows you to
see anyone

Since the goal of these two is to make healthcare more available and cost-effective, yet still of high quality

The Best Answer

(B) This is the best answer because it answers the question directly and presents a clear argument (based in fact) about why it is good for the profession.

The Mediocre Answer

(A) There are some good points in this answer (affordable care, for instance), and it is direct. However, the second part of the answer is not effective. First of all, it focuses blame for unethical treatment on physicians and shows you have a bias. It also gets away from the topic. And you didn't answer the question regarding impact on the profession.

The Weakest Answer

(C) Not only is this answer not necessarily correct, it does nothing to prove to the interviewers that you have given much thought to the issue. As was mentioned previously, you need to research issues related to health care so that you can effectively answer questions such as this.

31. "Do you think PAs and nurse practitioners are in competition with each other?"

Select the strongest answer.

A.) No. PAs and nurse practitioners have concern for the patient's well-being in common—just as physicians and nurses do. If we all work together to better the care for the patient, we all win in the end.

B.) No. PAs and nurse practitioners play different roles in the care of patients. PAs can prescribe medications, for instance, while nurse practitioners can't. Because our duties and responsibilities are different, we aren't in competition.

C.) No. PAs and nurse practitioners are both midlevel practitioners who fulfill a very important role in the health-care system. I look at both professions as working in collaboration as opposed to working against one another.

The Best Answer

(C) This is the best answer because it emphasizes the collaborative nature of patient care and the differing roles that individuals play within that collaboration.

The Mediocre Answer

(B) This answer begins to get at some of the differences and reasons why PAs and nurse practitioners are not in competition with each other, but it does not go in-depth enough. A better answer will address other differences and will show the interviewer that you have done your research.

The Weakest Answer

(A) This is the Miss America answer: world peace. While it sounds nice, it lacks depth and also a does not give the interviewers an idea of whether or not you actually do understand the differences between a PA and nurse practitioner.

32. "Where do PAs fit on the hierarchy ladder with nurses, MDs, and nurse practitioners?"

Select the strongest answer.

A.) PAs are higher in the hierarchy than nurses and nurse practitioners but lower than MDs.

B.) Technically, PAs are higher in the hierarchy than nurses and nurse practitioners but lower than MDs, but health care is all about team effort— so actually the hierarchy doesn't matter.

C.) We are all on the same team, so I don't necessarily think in terms of a hierarchy. Every team member, be it a nurse, physician, technician, or PA, has his or her own role and a common responsibility to provide the best care for the patient.

The Best Answer

(C) This answer is the best because it explains the collaborative nature of patient care and the importance of all members of the team working together.

The Mediocre Answer

(B) You have begun to address the power issues related to the hierarchy but fail to notice the nuanced issues associated with the hierarchy. The hierarchy does matter when it comes to directions and decisions regarding patient care.

The Weakest Answer

(A) This is the weakest answer because you aren't addressing the underlying power issues embedded in the question. While the order you list may be true, you've not talked about collaborative efforts and the teamwork associated with a health-care team.

33. "Is it important for PA students to belong to local, regional, and national PA associations? Why or why not?"

Select the strongest answer.

A.) Yes, it is very important. Belonging to a professional organization helps the PA make important networking contacts with others in the profession. It can also assist with job hunting and finding leads from others on job openings.

B.) Yes, it is important for many reasons. Professional organizations allow individuals to connect with others and learn about new trends in the field and also to support the profession.

C.) Yes. As medical professionals, it is important for PAs to remain current in both clinical and political issues at the state, regional, and national level. The profession is still a relatively new one, and PAs must remain vigilant concerning issues and policies in the health-care arena or risk negative consequences in the future.

The Best Answer

(C) In addition to giving the obvious "right" answer, you explain why you think it is important. The point about the profession being relatively new is important and shows critical thinking as well.

The Mediocre Answer

(B) You are on the right track here but need to expand your answer and get into the details of why it is important. This is your chance to show how you will give back to your field through your professional organization as well as why it is important for continuing education.

The Weakest Answer

(A) While you have the right answer (it is important), your reasons are all about you. It is important that you also talk about the educational potential of being a part of a regional and national organization.

Behavioral Questions

4

Most PA programs now utilize behavioral questions as their preferred way to choose top candidates, because they allow the interviewers to find out what specific skills, knowledge, and experience the PA school applicant possesses. What this means is that interviewers interpret what you say about yourself and your past behavior as an indicator of how you will behave in the future. In other words, if you did it before, you'll do it again. It is in your best interest to be able to demonstrate through the use of recent, relevant examples that you have done similar jobs with proven success.

While traditional questions ask you about something (e.g., How do you handle stress?), behavioral questions ask you to describe a specific situation and how you handled it (e.g., "Describe a very stressful situation you experienced and how you dealt with the stress in that situation?). Understand now that you will have tough behavioral questions in your interview.

Behavioral interview questions can be recognized by the wording used. A typical behavioral question might start with one of the following: "Tell me about…" Other examples include:

- "Can you give me an example…?"
- "Describe a time when…"
- "What was the biggest / most important / most difficult…?"
- "When was the…?"

As soon as you hear the interviewer asking for an example, you should start thinking about telling a "story" as proof that your background on paper supports your claims in real life. The key to answering behavioral questions is to be specific.

The more recent and medically related the example is, the more effective your answer will be.

If you don't have a recent, medically related example to relay, use a volunteer, college, or life experience. The important point is that in some way you relate to the qualities sought out in the question.

Remember these rules:

- Your examples must be specific.
- Your examples should be concise.
- Your examples should include action.
- Your examples must demonstrate your role.
- Your examples should be relevant to the questions asked.
- Your stories must have results.

HOW DO I PREPARE FOR A BEHAVIORAL INTERVIEW?

PA programs have a defined set of skills and "key competencies" they desire in PA students. These skill sets and competencies could include: decision making and problem solving, leadership, motivation, communication, interpersonal skills, critical thinking skills, the ability to work in a team, compassion, the ability to work autonomously, and the ability to influence others. These skill sets are based on the qualities and skills of a working physician assistant. In preparation for the PA school interview, the applicant should ask questions such as:

1. What are the necessary skills and "key competencies" to be a physician assistant?
2. What skills are necessary to be a physician assistant student?
3. What makes a successful PA school applicant?
4. What would make an unsuccessful applicant?
5. What is the most difficult part of being a physician assistant?

THE STAR TECHNIQUE

The best way to accomplish the goal of being specific is to use the three-step STAR process:

1. Situation or Task
2. Action
3. Result (or outcome)

For example, you may need to recall a time when you had to work under stressful conditions (situation). To handle the situation, you had to organize your employees and discuss options in order to accomplish the goal (action). Following the plan you developed, you were able to accomplish the goal (result). Using the three-step STAR process is a powerful way for you to frame your experiences.

Make sure you:

- Limit rambling and tangents. While you can't control what is asked, you can control what you say.
- Listen, listen, listen! Remember, we have two ears and one mouth for a reason. If you are unsure about what the question is, ask for clarification. When you respond, be sure to recall your past accomplishments in detail.
- Practice your behavioral strategies using real-life examples. It is very difficult to make up behavioral stories, which is why behavioral interviewing is becoming more popular. By practicing, you will be able to recall with confidence your past accomplishments.

Let's look at the following chart for help.

Situation or Task	Describe the situation that you were in or the task that you needed to accomplish. You must describe a specific event or situation, not a generalized description of what you have done in the past. Be sure to give enough detail for the interviewer to understand. The situation can be an event from a previous job or from a volunteer experience or any relevant event.
Action You Took	Describe the action you took, and be sure to keep the focus on you. Even if you are discussing a group project or effort, describe what you did—not the efforts of the team. Don't tell what you might do, tell what you did.
Results You Achieved	What happened? How did the event end? What did you accomplish? What did you learn?

Use examples from internships, classes, school projects, activities, team participation, community service, hobbies, and work experience—anything really—as examples of your past behavior. In addition, you may use examples of special accomplishments, whether personal or professional, such as scoring the winning touchdown, being elected to office in your Italian organization, winning a prize for your artwork, surfing a big wave, or raising money for charity. Wherever possible, quantify your results. Numbers always impress committee members.

Remember that many behavioral questions try to get at how you responded to negative situations; you'll need to have examples of negative experiences ready, but try to choose negative experiences that you made the best of—better yet, those that had positive outcomes.

Here's a good way to prepare for behavior-based interviews:

- Identify six to eight examples from your past experience where you demonstrated top behaviors and skills that PA school admissions committees seek.
- Half your examples should be totally positive, like accomplishments or meeting goals.
- The other half should be situations that started out negatively but either ended positively or you made the best of the outcome.
- Vary your examples; don't take them all from just one area of your life.
- Use fairly recent examples. If you are a college student, examples from high school may be too long ago. Try to select examples from the past year.
- Try to describe examples in story form or use the STAR technique.

To prepare for the behavioral interview, the night before you're interviewed, review your CASPA application and your résumé. Seeing your achievements in print will jog your memory. In the interview, listen carefully to each question, and pull an example out of your bag of tricks that provides an appropriate description of how you demonstrated the desired behavior. With practice, you can learn to tailor a relatively small set of examples to respond to a number of different behavioral questions.

Ready to practice? Let's get started.

BEHAVIORAL QUESTIONS AND ANSWERS

1. "Tell me about a time when you had to overcome obstacles to get your job done?"

Select the strongest answer.

A.) When I was a navy corpsman on a field maneuver in Brandisi, Italy, we had a mock battle with the Italian Marines. The battle took place on rough terrain, and we suffered multiple casualties, from sprained ankles to a separated shoulder. In the field, corpsman carried all of their supplies in a small bag about the size of a medium-sized purse. We quickly ran out of ACE wraps and bandages. We also had the problem of the patient with a separated shoulder. As my unit's medical person, I had to call in a medevac to get the marine with the shoulder injury back to the ship, and I had to utilize my limited Italian to ask the Italian Marines for extra supplies. It all worked out in the end, and we accomplished the mission.

B.) I have to work around obstacles all of the time. It's the nature of the job as a medical assistant. One day, I have to work around time constraints; the next day, it's schedules and deadlines. Of course, I always have people problems to contend with. Every day, I plan my day, and then, right when I am getting ahead, some problem occurs. Fortunately, I look at problems as opportunities.

C.) I have had many instances in jobs when I have had to put in overtime to solve problems that have come up. One thing I try always to do is think logically and stay focused. I can usually handle anything that comes my way. I had times when a whole project depended on me to get it out the door on time. I came through with flying colors. My supervisor is sometimes amazed at what I can accomplish.

The Strongest Answer

(A) This is the only answer of the three that addresses the question asked. The question begins, "Tell me about a time…" Whenever you are asked about "a time," the interviewer is looking for a specific example. This answer shows that you handled the crisis, how you did it, and the results of your efforts.

The Mediocre Answer

(C) This is not a bad answer, but it doesn't answer the question. It is very general and needs to be more specific. You provide a lot of good qualities in this answer, but there is no specific example. Anyone can say, "I can handle anything that comes my way," but the interviewer is looking for an example of when you actually did that.

The Weakest Answer

(B) This answer is very nonspecific. It is very general and does not provide an example of "a time when" you had to overcome an obstacle. It would be a much stronger answer if it included specific details of how and when you solved a problem. The tone of this answer could also be a problem. An interviewer might read between the lines and pick up on the idea that you are "burned-out" on this work.

2. "Tell me about a time when you had to handle a stressful situation?"

Select the strongest answer.

A.) That's the way life is in the emergency room. We always seem to be short-staffed. If you can't handle the stress, you can't succeed as a nurse. We all work as hard as we can and as fast as we can, but sometimes that's just not enough. We get complaints and have to deal with it. I have had instances where I have had as many as twenty patients and had to handle it. That's just the nature of the game. I am good at what I do, and I do whatever it takes to get the job done. There are always shortages and budget problems, and you just have to deal with it. I have what is needed to do the job.

B.) I was a fresh, new lieutenant assigned to the 554th Range Group at Nellis Air Force Base, Nevada. One of my first assignments was to go 250 miles north of Las Vegas to a bombing range in the desert. This range was used by fighter pilots from all over the world to practice aerial tactics and bomb ground targets built out of plywood. I was in charge of "Coronet Clean," a range cleanup operation that included carpenters, explosive ordnance disposal personnel, and other noncommissioned officers. Our job was to clear the range of unexploded bombs, rebuild the blown-up targets, and do it safely and quickly. This was not easy, as every piece of plywood harbored a sidewinder rattlesnake underneath it, and I'm terrified of snakes. Although I had no expertise in any of these areas, I met with my senior noncommissioned officers every morning to make a plan for the day. I stayed I touch with my people and headquarters via telecommunications. We accomplished the goal ahead of time and received a letter of commendation for our efforts.

C.) I know what it takes to get the job done. I pride myself on staying calm when everything around me is falling apart. I don't like stress, but know how to deal with it. I just do my work and try to ignore unpleasant things that take place. I'm paid to do a service, and I do it. We each have our own area of responsibility. I do mine, and I do it well. I get through my shift, and that's the end. I don't take problems home with me.

The Strongest Answer

(B) This is the strongest answer because it provides an example of a real team player handling stressful situations. This reply demonstrates by example the ability to remain cool and think straight when things are too hot to handle. The skills and attributes evident in this example are teamwork, adaptability, the ability to handle pressure, the ability to prioritize, a sense of humor, and the ability to communicate.

The Mediocre Answer

(A) This is not the strongest answer, but it does have merit. It does not give a specific example, which we asked for in the question. It would be a stronger answer if it was expanded with a specific example. The statement "I've had as many as twenty patients" shows the scope of responsibility, but a specific example would have shown the skills it took to deal with the situation.

The Weakest Answer

(C) This is the weakest answer. In addition to sounding negative, it does not address the question about a specific time. This answer has the tone of someone with a defeatist attitude. That may be the way things are, but the answer points out all the negatives of the job and none of the positives. This answer could be interpreted as coming from a person who is burned-out or has given up trying to improve the situation.

3. "Tell me about a time when you had to adapt quickly to a change?"

Select the strongest answer.

A.) I was working as a phlebotomist in a primary-care clinic, when we had a major flu epidemic hit our area. Three of our medical assistants called in sick for the week. Prior to becoming a phlebotomist, I worked as a certified medical assistant. I immediately had to wear two hats—that of a medical assistant and that of a phlebotomist. I called patients who were scheduled for blood draws and coordinated their appointments for specific times at a slower pace during the week. I worked extremely hard that week multitasking, but we maintained our patient volume and had not one complaint about waiting times.

B.) I actually like change. In fact, I thrive on change. I am a person who can adapt to any situation you put me in. I worked for one internal medicine practice where the office manager changed three times in one year. I didn't let it get to me. I am flexible and roll with the punches. Some people are like oak trees that don't bend very much and will break in a storm. I am more like a palm tree; I go with the flow and bend without breaking. I like being challenged.

C.) Change is inevitable. The only certainty in life is change. Change can be frustrating and terrifying at times, but that's how we know we're changing! But change has been really frustrating lately at my current job. There were just too many changes, without any thought behind them. I don't want to complain about management, but sometimes they changed the way we were doing something and the week later changed it back to the way it had been before. That can be very frustrating for an employee.

The Strongest Answer

(A) This is the strongest answer because it gives a very action-oriented example. There was a problem. You moved quickly to solve the problem. The problem was resolved. There is a strong sense of what your role was in the situation. This answer also would be a good reply to a question dealing with problem solving or coming up with a creative idea.

The Mediocre Answer

(B) This answer is not as strong as (A), but it is fairly creative with a great analogy about the "palm tree" and the "oak tree." However, it would be much better with a specific example of how you dealt with a particular problem and resolved it.

The Weakest Answer

(C) This answer has a negative, whiny tone. It is not a good idea to badmouth former employers in an interview. Even if there were negative circumstances, it is best to let it go in the interview.

4. "Your application states that you're a 'hard worker.' Can you give me an example of a time when you worked hard?"

Select the strongest answer.

A.) I always try to get the work done on time. Sometimes that means working overtime. Sometimes I can't get all my work done during the day and am willing to stay late to finish up. There have been times when I just couldn't get everything done, no matter how hard I worked. I always do my best to meet deadlines, but sometimes you just have to let go. I'd rather do it right and be late than do it wrong and be on time.

B.) I am a very hard worker. I am always punctual and get my work done. The tighter the deadline is, the harder I work. I plan my day so that I'm never late with my work, and I always meet deadlines. If you ask my last boss, he will tell you what a hard worker I am. I do whatever I have to do to get the job done.

C.) My boss had a really important project, and it didn't look like we were going to make the deadline. I volunteered to do some late nights and weekends. My boss and two other co-workers worked seven straight days with no time off. My piece of the project was to coordinate all the information and enter the data. It was a real team effort, but we were able to meet the deadline, and that made my boss look good. He rewarded us all for our efforts.

The Strongest Answer

(C) This is the strongest answer because it gives a specific example of going "above and beyond" what was expected. Some of the skills that appear in this answer are initiative, teamwork, coordination skills, a great attitude, and a cooperative spirit—and a willingness to make the boss look good.

The Mediocre Answer

(B) This is not as strong an answer. It provides all the right traits—punctuality, conscientiousness, good attitude—but no examples of using those traits in an actual situation. This answer does not benefit from the endorsement from your boss. Bringing the boss into the story is a great way to strengthen the story though.

The Weakest Answer

(A) This is the weakest answer because it does not include an example of working hard and emphasizes meeting deadlines, which is not quite the same skill. The interviewer could get the idea that you miss deadlines and have a difficult time keeping up with the workload. This answer needs to emphasize the times you stayed late and why the workload was too big to handle.

5. "Describe an interaction you've had with a patient that made an impact on you."

Select the strongest answer.

A.) I've had many patients impact me in a variety of ways. I always come away humbled by the experience of how health-care providers can help a very ill person become well. I've found that medicine isn't just about IVs, antibiotics, and pills. Rather, good medicine comes from the heart and feelings of the caregiver. Working in medicine is a true calling and one that I look forward to pursuing as a PA.

B.) I can't choose just one patient who's had a major impact on me. I work as an emergency room technician, and we see a variety of patients on a daily basis. Most of the time these patients are in the acute phase of an illness or injury, and the best I can do is hold their hand and tell them everything is going to be okay. The patients appreciate this, and it makes me feel good that I can play a small part in their recovery. I know as a PA, I will be able to play a more significant and advanced role in the diagnosing and treating of my patients.

C.) Susie was an IV drug abuser having her third mitral valve replacement. I was shadowing a cardiothoracic surgery PA and was able to be in the OR for her surgery. I recall the surgeon and his first assistant talking about the patient's lifestyle during the procedure. The talk was really negative and centered on her drug abuse and the fact that she was killing herself. I felt the conversation was inappropriate, but as an "invited guest," I was not going to make any comments. The surgery went fine, but as I made rounds with the PA later that day, the patient confronted him. She said, "I heard everything you all said about me in there. I know I have a drug problem, but I'm not a bad person." I learned a valuable lesson that day. Never judge patients for their lifestyle choices. That's not our job. Also, don't gossip about patients; it's rude and unprofessional.

The Strongest Answer

(C) This is a powerful example of a lesson learned and a memorable patient. The answer is believable in the fact that you would probably never again talk about a patient, whether the patient is unconscious or behind the next curtain. There is a lesson here for all providers of health care. The answer also shows your good judgment in not saying anything during the procedure; that would be inappropriate unless you were actually a medical provider responsible for the care of that patient. As an observer, you did the right thing.

The Mediocre Answer

(B) This answer is the next best because it shows your compassion, but it does not provide a specific example of a patient who "made an impact on you." Remember to answer the question! The hand-holding gesture is a good example of how to comfort someone, but a specific example would have made this answer much more interesting.

The Weakest Answer

(A) This is the weakest answer because it doesn't even come close to answering the question. In fact, the interviewer will get the feeling that you have not had much patient care experience after hearing this one.

6. "Tell me about a time when you had a disagreement or confrontation with a boss or co-worker."

Select the strongest answer.

A.) My boss refused to take action against an employee who was getting away with something that went against company policy. I was upset about the situation. I feel that everyone should be treated equally, and it was wrong for this person to get away with something when the rest of us had to conform. I talked to my boss, but that didn't work. I ended up going to human resources and complaining. My boss was unhappy with me for going over his head, but action was taken and the employee was disciplined. My boss eventually got over it.

B.) I'm one of those people who try to get along with everyone. I try to ignore people who have irritating qualities. I believe we have to choose our battles, so to speak. I try to be as professional as possible when I work. If I get upset, I go for a walk or take a break to get away from the situation. I really don't like confrontation.

C.) There was a co-worker who was taking extra time off at lunch and giving me a problem because I was her backup. Rather than let it fester, I asked her if we could talk after work. I explained to her in a civil manner that there was a problem. She told me that she had been trying to accomplish personal tasks at lunch that were taking longer than expected and that she would stop doing that. She hadn't thought about the impact it was having on my work. Things changed for the better after our discussion.

The Strongest Answer

(C) This is the strongest answer. Communication skills are the most important skills in most professions. This answer demonstrates the ability to face up to difficult situations and "nip the problem" before it becomes full-blown.

The Mediocre Answer

(A) This is a good answer because it is specific, but it is a bit risky to give an example of a time when you went against your boss. This incident had a positive result, but if you were interviewing with a PA who happened to be a supervisor as well, it might cause some doubt about your ability to cooperate as an employee. It would be advisable to stay away from stories that make your boss look weak, especially if you are interviewing with a boss.

The Weakest Answer

(B) This isn't a bad answer, but it is somewhat passive, as demonstrated in the phrases "I try to ignore people," "If I get upset, I go for a walk," and "I really don't like confrontation." The interviewer might be thinking, *As a PA, you are going to be taking a lot of walks!*

7. "You mentioned in your essay that you are 'good at selling new ideas to your boss and co-workers.' How do you do that?"

Select the strongest answer.

A.) My current boss is not very receptive to new ideas. I was able to sell her on one of my ideas when I showed her a work schedule that would optimize our coverage on the weekend shifts. Behind the scenes, I put together a lot of data and analysis that included details, facts, and figures. That extra effort really paid off when I presented her with the idea. She is one of those people who needs facts to make decisions. She trusted me a lot more after that.

B.) My boss would tell you that I am always selling him on ideas. I have at least one idea a week. Some work; some don't. My success rate is about 75 percent positive. One of the frustrations that I have is getting through the hospital hierarchy. When you work for a large institution, it can sometimes take weeks to get an idea through the mill. I am an action-oriented guy who wants to make things happen. Sometimes it takes so long to get an idea through the channels that it is less effective than it would be if I had been able to start it when I first had the idea.

C.) I figured out a way for our clinic to see more patients in less time by using a different scheduling practice. I met with my boss to convince her of my idea, and she reluctantly gave me the go-ahead. I then met with the office manager, CEO, and medical director. Working together, we tweaked the plan and refined some of the bottleneck areas of our clinic. I calculated the new amount of patient volume we could handle, as well as the potential increased patient satisfaction and presented it to my boss for her approval. I really surprised her with the numbers and my 30 percent increase in patient volume. She approved the plan. The best part was the patient satisfaction survey that showed a significant improvement in perceived wait times and ability to get appointments sooner.

The Strongest Answer

(C) This is the strongest answer because of the clear example it gives of action on your part. You laid the steps out: the situation, the action you took, the results. Showing a positive outcome makes for a good success story. There are times, however, when the outcome may not be positive for the company for reasons that are completely out of your control. When this is the case, keep the focus on your role in the project and the way you completed your task. Do not dwell on the company's problems. This is about you and the skills you have to offer. Talk about what you were responsible for and how your part was finished successfully even if there were no positive results. An example would be a project that was shelved after you did all the work to complete it.

The Mediocre Answer

(A) This is not a bad answer, but it could be strengthened by more detail. Describing the analytic process and the types of facts and figures that you found and presented would be more effective. The good parts of this story are your ability to understand that your boss has a style, which requires facts, and your ability to adapt your approach to meet her needs.

The Weakest Answer

(B) This answer is too general; it provides no facts. It also presents the complaining side of dealing with the process, which may or may not occur in the new job. It is best to ask questions about the process first and then judge whether your role in a new culture is going to be different from the one you left.

8. "Tell me about a time when your communication skills made a difference?"

Select the strongest answer.

A.) I have strong written and verbal communication skills. I write a great deal of the protocols for our x-ray department teaching programs. I've worked with great teams and focused on the invaluable role of focus groups as a source of improving our curriculum. I have written interactive exercises and developed creative test models that are used as standards in the department's program for x-ray students. Communication with the teams I have worked with has made a huge difference in the success of my projects. I couldn't have done it without their cooperation and communication.

B.) I have over five years of experience developing and delivering programs for EMT training courses. I develop, organize, and conduct educational seminars all over the state of Texas, focusing on preparing students for their exams. I helped produce a series of DVDs that support the material I teach. I am known for my passionate delivery and presentation of materials that have been viewed as boring and uninteresting when presented by others. It's the way you present the information that makes the difference.

C.) One project that I worked on involved developing the curriculum for a program dealing with cultural similarities in everyday life. The challenge was to communicate with my team members and get them as excited about their roles in the project as I was about mine. I talked to them individually, drawing out the particular interests they had. I used this information to assign responsibility where there was interest, enabling me to bring about extremely positive results through a team effort. The feedback from the team was that every person felt he or she had made a contribution in his or her own special way. It was worth the extra effort I made to listen and obtain their input.

The Strongest Answer

(C) This is the strongest answer because of the way you used communication skills to work with individuals, listening and implementing the ideas you heard. Because good communication skills require listening and writing as well as speaking, you have demonstrated a broad use of your skills. This is an answer that also shows strong leadership skills as well as the ability to appreciate the differences people bring to a situation.

The Mediocre Answer

(A) This answer has all the makings of a good story; it just needs to be rearranged to focus on the communication issues and address the question. If you compare this example with the stronger answer (C), you can see how the same information is there, but (C) places more emphasis on communication with the team, which brought about successful results.

The Weakest Answer

(B) This answer speaks about your experiences as they are written on your application, not as a relevant example of your experience. A specific example of any one of the skills you mentioned would be stronger than reiterating your application content. The last part of this answer could be developed as an example of your presentation to a group and the feedback you obtained about your passionate delivery.

9. "Give me an example of a time when you took initiative."

Select the strongest answer.

A.) When I took over the department in my last job, there were turnover problems. I sat down with the staff members and asked them why so many people were leaving. I learned that when they were hired, they were told that there would be cross-functional training, and it never happened. I consider my team to be my main customer, and I immediately set a plan into motion. It involved presenting my plan to my manager and requesting extra time and money. I put my job on the line, but I got what we needed. I turned the department around and bought some strong loyalty from my staff.

B.) I attempted to initiate things in my last company, but nobody was really interested in what I had to say. I always volunteer and am always glad to help in any way that I can, but I don't want to take the responsibility for initiating projects. The last time I initiated something for a company, I got stuck with all the responsibility and work. I gave up trying to do something other than my job. Don't get me wrong. I am a hard worker and am more than willing to pull my weight, but I let other people lead.

C.) This is an example from my life outside my job, but it is a project that I am very proud of. I was responsible for initiating a clothing drive for the homeless in our city. It came about when we were talking at lunch one day. There is a woman who hangs out near our building, and we felt sorry for her because it was getting cold. Some of us had clothes and blankets that we were glad to donate, but we didn't know exactly how to approach the situation. I volunteered to research the situation and set up a drive. Some of my co-workers volunteered to help. By the end of the month, we had collected so many coats and blankets that we presented them to the city for the shelters. We got a commendation from the mayor.

The Strongest Answer

(A) This is the strongest answer because it gives a good example of stepping up to the plate and initiating action—getting things done. This is a strong example of being a good leader who takes the time to listen and respond. It is also an answer that shows strong qualities for motivating others and handling groups.

The Mediocre Answer

(C) This is not a bad answer. If you don't have a work-related experience to talk about, talking about a volunteer or personal situation is reasonable as long as it is appropriate in regard to the question. In this case, you took the initiative to set up and research a program to help others.

The Weakest Answer

(B) This is the weakest answer because of the tone more than the content. It sounds negative and angry. It's not so much what is said but the impression it gives. If you don't want to lead, that is acceptable. But try to focus on the positive side of what you've done in the interview. Negative attitudes are a real turnoff for interviewers.

10. "Have you ever been in a situation, at work or in school, where you felt it was necessary to address an ethical issue? Describe that situation."

Select the strongest answer.

A.) When I was a sophomore in college, I took a class in which we had to do group work. While most members of the group worked equally hard on the project, one member was a loafer and didn't do a thing. At the end of the term, the professor asked us to evaluate one another in the group, and this particular student asked us all to give him a good evaluation in spite of the fact that he didn't do much work. Some said they would, but I refused to give him a good evaluation because I didn't think it was fair. He already got a good grade on our group project and now he wanted a good grade on participation.

B.) When I was working as a nursing assistant, I suspected that another nursing assistant was not changing the bed position of a patient who needed to be turned every two hours. I had cared for that patient the previous day, and I knew he was in pretty bad shape and most likely would die. Because patient care is my number-one concern, I asked the other nursing assistant if she needed help with the patient (even though I wasn't assigned to him). I told her that I had cared for him the previous day, and I knew that he needed special attention. While she told me that she didn't need help, I did notice that she immediately began to attend to him more thoughtfully—most likely because she knew I was watching out for him.

C.) When I was working in the pharmaceutical industry, I experienced many examples of unethical study methods used by employees of my company in drug testing. It always made me a bit uncomfortable to know that this was going on. It was all about the profits.

The Strongest Answer

(B) This is the strongest answer because it emphasizes many good qualities—concern for the patient, a willingness to take a risk and confront a co-worker who isn't caring for the patient, and creativity and sensibility in managing this conflict.

The Mediocre Answer

(A) This situation could be a great situation to discuss because you are talking about issues associated with teamwork. Clearly, effective teamwork is a critical component of health care. You missed the opportunity to talk about that with this answer.

The Weakest Answer

(C) This answer is not good because while you bring up the problem, you don't talk about the solution. You leave the interviewer with the impression that while you are "a bit uncomfortable" with unethical practices, you don't have the courage to do anything about it or to change it.

11. "If you and a colleague had a personality clash, what would you do to make it better?"

Select the strongest answer.

A.) It depends upon the importance of the clash. If it wasn't a big deal, I'd just ignore it and hope it went away. If it created a bigger problem, I would probably wait a while and then try to sit down with the person and talk about it.

B.) I tend to be a conflict avoider, so I would probably just let it go. In the big scheme of life, most personality clashes are not that big of a deal.

C.) If I could, I would wait a bit and give each of us time to cool off. I think perspective is important, and sometimes waiting gives people a chance to see the other person's side of the issue. Then I would ask to talk with the person and find a time that works. I would discuss the problem with him or her and try to come to a good solution. If I couldn't wait and the issue needed to be resolved immediately, I would take a breath to calm myself and then try to discuss it with the other person. I would try to get to a win-win solution so that each of us was satisfied with the outcome.

The Strongest Answer

(C) This is the strongest answer because you display good understanding of conflict and conflict resolution. You acknowledge the fact that parties in a conflict need to cool off and that trying to find a win-win solution is the best way to approach a conflict.

The Mediocre Answer

(A) While it probably is a good answer in that you have thought a bit about the magnitude of the conflict and the extent to which it needs to be addressed, you've failed to discuss how personality differences can impact health-care teams and ultimately patient care.

The Weakest Answer

(B) This answer has a negative, whiny tone. It is not a good idea to badmouth former employers in an interview. Even if there were negative circumstances, it is best to let it go in the interview.

12. "Do you think it's important to promote team building in an organization? What steps will you take as a PA student to promote team building in the class?"

Select the strongest answer.

A.) Yes, I think team building should be promoted in organizations. Part of learning in a classroom environment is learning from other students. Collaborative teamwork improves learning. I would do at least three things to promote teamwork in the class. First, I would be a good team member. Second, I would promote social interaction in the class because social relationships promote team relationships. Third, I would encourage classmates to confront conflicts directly and resolve them as soon as possible. It important for us to learn about teamwork in our schooling since much of what we will be doing as a PA is working in a collaborative team environment.

B.) Team building is critical to most organizations. So I do think it is very important. First, I would promote team building in the class by being a good team member. Second, I like to organize social events, so I would do that for the class to add some social dynamic to the class and help with cohesion.

C.) Yes, team building is important in organizations. But so is working alone. I personally think that team building is emphasized too much in more organizations today. The value of the individual is downplayed. When dealing with patients, many decisions are individual and teams often don't work effectively so that is a good thing.

new ideas
prepares you for working
in a team in a hospital
or clinic setting

The Strongest Answer

(A) This is the strongest answer because the response specifically addresses the question by telling the interviewer what you would do to build teamwork in the class and also talks about why this is important for the field.

The Mediocre Answer

(B) This answer is not as strong as (A), but it is a good response because you acknowledge the importance of team building and also give a couple of ideas for how you would help build teams in the class. You could, however, do much more with this answer by talking about the importance of teams to the profession and the ways in which student and class team building will positively impact your work as a PA.

The Weakest Answer

(C) This answer is negative and contradictory. While you say it is important, you spend the rest of the time talking about how individual action is important. An answer like this would be a red flag to an interviewer who may see you as someone unable to work effectively on teams.

13. "From your perspective, describe what makes a person 'likeable'?"

Select the strongest answer.

A.) (A) Being friendly is very important to being likeable. Research shows that people tend to like people who like them, so friendliness is important. Being genuine and being a good listener are also important. Finally, and perhaps most important for being successful as a PA, individuals who are empathic are liked. Patients need to know that their health-care provider cares about them and to a certain degree, understands their problems and can relate to their pain (physical or emotional).

B.) (B) I actually think that likeability is something you either have or you don't have. I guess I would say it is similar to charisma—some people have it, and others don't.

C.) (C) I think the following things make people likeable: a nice smile, a willingness to listen to others, good grooming (you need not be beautiful but well groomed), and the ability to engage in small talk.

The Strongest Answer

(A) This is the strongest answer because it shows that you know what likeability is all about and gets at why it is important for a PA to be likeable.

The Mediocre Answer

(C) This answer starts to get at some important aspects of likeability, but you don't go far enough to describe why these qualities make someone likeable. You would also want to talk about why likeability is important to being a PA.

The Weakest Answer

(B) This is a weak answer because it gives the interviewer no real information about what you believe to be important in likeability (aside from the elusive concept of "charisma").

Ethical Questions

5

WHAT ARE ETHICAL ISSUES?

Ethical issues are problems or dilemmas involving moral compromise. They can arise anywhere. They can be thought of on a societal scale, like, "Should gays be allowed to marry?" or on an individual level, like, "Does a priest have the right to refuse marrying a same-sex couple?"

During the course of your PA school interview(s), you are very likely to be asked one or more ethical questions as they relate to health care. The following topics are a typical source of medical ethical questions:

- Abortion
- Managed care
- Patient confidentiality
- Refusal and withdrawal of treatment
- Genetic testing
- Medical malpractice
- Professional ethics

THE EIGHT MOST COMMON ETHICAL SCENARIOS

1) "If you had to choose to give a transplant either to a successful elderly member of the community or a twenty-year-old drug addict, which would you choose?"

This is a common PA school interview question, and your initial response may be something like this: It is not in my power to determine the value of human life. I would defer to the waiting list protocol.

However, if you don't make a choice, you are not really answering the question. If you want to give an effective answer, you have to choose; you don't get to opt out of making a choice on this one.

I would choose the elderly patient who is a productive member of society and who has done nothing to compromise his or her health and is most likely to have a successful transplant.

The drug addict will not even make it to the transplant list if he or she has not been clean for a designated period of time. Additionally, after the transplant, patients need to be extremely responsible with follow-up visits, medication regimens, and maintaining a healthy lifestyle.

(Note that you are not making a judgment on the drug addict, you are simply stating the facts of the situation.)

2) "A patient of yours was recently diagnosed with HIV, and he demands that you don't tell his wife because he fears she will leave him. His wife is also your patient. What will you tell her?"

This is a very common ethical scenario that may be presented to you at a PA school interview. This scenario relates to *patient confidentiality*.

As a medical provider, you should always do your best to respect patient privacy. However, the patient's right to privacy is not unconditional. Confidentiality may be legally breached in five special circumstances:

1. The court orders you to do so;
2. The patient gives permission to release information;
3. There is the possibility of harm to vulnerable persons (child abuse, elder abuse);
4. It is in the interest of public welfare, as with reporting sexually transmitted diseases to the health department;
5. A third party is threatened, as with a patient divulging a murder plan.

In the above scenario, public welfare is the issue, and once you report the HIV-positive status to the health department, they will approach the wife.

3. "A patient is admitted to the intensive care unit with severe coronary artery disease. The patient is a Jehovah's Witness and declares that he cannot receive any form of blood products because of his religious beliefs. Immediately after the sur-

gery, the patient begins bleeding severely from 'everywhere.' Without the blood products, he is likely to die. What are your options?"

This scenario concerns "refusal and withdrawal of treatment." Patients have the
right to make their own health-care decisions, and medical providers have the obligation to honor those decisions. Patients who are competent can start, stop, or refuse
treatment. The medical provider's responsibility in this scenario is to disclose the
consequences of not taking the treatment.

As with informed consent, with treatment refusal, practitioners are responsible
for giving full disclosure of relevant medical information and allowing free and effective decision-making by patients. They must also determine competence and respect
patient personal, religious, and cultural values.

4. "You are a PA working in a cardiology practice. Although you attend to the
majority of the patients in a typical day, your supervising physician signs all of the
charts and assigns the medical billing codes. You notice that he is coding higher for
Medicare and Medicaid patients because, 'We don't get reimbursed enough.' You are
concerned that you may have some liability if the physician gets caught overbilling
(fraud). What do you do?"

The supervising physician is clearly billing Medicare and Medicaid at higher
levels than indicated; thus he is committing Medicare and Medicaid *fraud*.

The medical code of ethics obliges you to report incompetence, impairment, or
misconduct of your colleagues. As a medical provider you "…shall…report to the
appropriate authorities those physicians who practice unethically or incompetently or
who engage in fraud or deception."[6]

Reporting your supervising physician to the authorities is certainly easier said
than done. After all, this person is paying your salary. However, you do not have to
go from "zero to sixty" without stopping in between. Reporting your supervising
physician should be your last resort.

The first step may be to have a discussion with him. Describe the situation and
explain how you feel about it. Next, assert yourself by telling him that you are not
willing to risk your career over such practices. Finally, ask the physician for a solution
to the problem. If you are able to work out a solution with your supervising physician, the matter need not go any further.

If not, you may need to take the matter to the next level. If you work in a group
practice, you can approach the senior partners or the CEO. If you cannot resolve
the matter at this level, you are obliged to report your concerns to the appropriate
authorities or risk criminal/legal liability.

---

6   WMA International Code of Medical Ethics

5. "Do you believe that all individuals have a right to health care in this country?"

A "right" to health care is actually an "entitlement" right. Entitlement rights are limited by a society's willingness and ability to provide the entitlement. In the United States, entitlements depend on financial resources and the decisions we make on how to best utilize those resources.

Even if you think health care is a right, how could we provide the highest level of medical care to everyone? We would certainly have to address the idea of some form of rationing, and who, then, would determine the minimum allotment?

As medical providers, it is our duty and obligation to treat every patient to the best of our ability. It is not up to us to determine who qualifies for that treatment. Those decisions are largely left up to the politicians and insurance companies. To this end, our hands are somewhat tied.

6. "You catch your colleague stealing restricted drugs. She says, 'Please don't tell anyone. I'm doing this to help a friend who doesn't have the money and insurance to pay.' What would you do?"

Stealing controlled medication is a criminal offense. Clearly, you could not turn your back and ignore the situation. You would state the facts to your colleague, telling her that she is stealing controlled medication for a friend and that is an illegal and punishable offense. You should then tell her that she is also placing you in a position of liability and that you are not willing to assume that liability for her actions. Finally, you should tell your colleague that if she doesn't bring this up to your supervisor, you will.

7. "What would you do if you were a PA in the emergency department, and the paramedics wheeled in a patient whom you found out just stabbed your best friend?"

Although you would be extremely emotional and perhaps very angry, it is your obligation to treat every patient to the best of your ability. You should not refuse to treat the patient, unless you are too emotional to be effective. Then you simply ask one of your colleagues to take over for you.

8. "How do you feel about abortion? Would you assist a physician in performing abortions?"

Deciding to have an abortion is a very personal and complex issue. I personally believe that every abortion should be considered on a case-by-case basis. Abortion has been legal in every state since 1973 (*Roe v. Wade*). As long as abortion is legal, women have the right to choose.

If you decided to work in a practice where abortions are performed, you would clearly have made a choice to assist in abortions.

However, I stand firm on the fact that medical providers have a duty and an obligation to provide the best quality of health care to our patients, no matter what the circumstances.

Situational Questions

6

Responses to situational questions can make or break an interview. An interviewer uses situational interviewing techniques to elicit specific examples of an applicant's ability to perform under stress, work as a team player, and communicate with physicians and other health-care professionals. Additionally, the interviewer will want to determine how well you understand the role of the PA.

As the interviewer finds out more about you and the way you behave in certain situations, you begin generating a profile of your skill sets, attitudes, and ability to deal with a variety of situations.

A successful situational interview question response tells a good story. Key point: if you are asked a question that begins with "Describe a situation when…" or "Tell me about a time when…" or "Can you give me an example…" you should immediately think "story."

TARGET YOUR AUDIENCE

Telling a story consists of relating an incident or telling about an experience you've had through a vignette (short tale or story). In order to do this effectively, you must always keep your audience in mind, which will be PAs, PA students, and faculty of the PA program. Your goal is to create interest and desire by telling a story. This section will focus on techniques to make your vignettes compelling and effective.

THE ELEMENTS OF YOUR STORY

The elements that go into a good story include a beginning, middle, and an end. By following the simple technique of including these elements, you will make it much easier for the interviewer to follow your stories. This is important because you want to make an emotional connection with the interviewer, and you do this with eye contact and open gestures and by maintaining the attention of the person interviewing you.

Here are three rules to follow:

1. Have a strong beginning—State the problem.
2. Support your beginning with a strong middle—What was your role in solving the problem?
3. Provide a strong end to the story—What was the result?

Let's examine a sample question:
"Tell me about a time when you had to handle a stressful situation?"
Step 1: The task is to tell the interviewer about a "stressful" situation and how you "had to handle" it. So you must first start by stating "the problem."

The Beginning:

I was a fresh, new lieutenant assigned to the 554th Range Group at Nellis Air Force Base, Nevada. One of my first assignments was to travel 250 miles north of Las Vegas to a bombing range in the desert. This range was used by fighter pilots from all over the world, in an exercise called "Red Flag," to practice aerial tactics and bomb ground targets built out of plywood. We also had live operations going on at different parts of the range.

Here, the answer is clear, concise, and may even get the interviewer to lean a little forward in his or her chair to hear the rest.

Step 2: Next, include action steps to make it very clear to the interviewer what you did to resolve the problem. What were the exact steps that you took?

The Middle:

I was in charge of "Coronet Clean," a range cleanup operation that includes carpenters, explosive ordnance disposal (EOD) personnel, and other noncommissioned officers (NCOs). Our job was to clear the range of unexploded bombs, rebuild the blown-up targets, and do this safely and quickly. This was not easy, as every piece of plywood harbored a sidewinder rattlesnake underneath it, and I'm terrified of snakes.

Although I had no expertise in any of these areas, I met with my senior noncommissioned officers every morning to make a plan for the day. I touched base with the EOD people to see where they would be clearing bombs. I touched base with the carpenters, to see where they would be rebuilding targets. I stayed in touch with the senior NCOs and headquarters at Nellis Air Force Base, via telecommunications, to be sure the range wasn't going to be used during the times we were working.

The interviewee is painting a good picture of the task and the stress involved. More important, he demonstrates his specific role in getting this job accomplished.

The End:

We accomplished the goal ahead of time, with no casualties, and our unit received a letter of commendation for our efforts. I felt proud that I was a part of that mission.

This is a straight, to-the-point answer that had a definitive and positive outcome. The goal was accomplished on time, with no casualties, and the interviewee received a letter of commendation.

The interviewer will gain from this story knowing that you can handle stress under fire (literally) and that you will probably be able to do this again in other situations.

EXERCISE: WHAT'S YOUR STORY?

Obviously, the above example is very effective. If you are a veteran, you can probably come up with many similar stories. But what if you've never been in the military?

What if you're just graduating college? How do you come up with, or compete with, a story like that?

The good news is that you don't have to have such a dramatic story. You just need to come up with an answer that will be of interest to the interviewer.

For this exercise, identify a situation or problem you have faced which you were able resolve, feel good about, and received praise for.

Follow the three-step plan outlined above:

Step 1: Beginning—What was the problem?
Step 2: Middle—What did you do about the problem?
Step 3: End—How did it turn out?

TELL YOUR STORY: PROPORTIONS

The beginning of your story should take about 20 percent or less of your time and focus on the situation, task, or problem.

The middle of the story should consume 60 percent or more and includes the action, the steps taken to solve the problem, the ideas generated, the tasks performed, and the challenges you overcame to successfully accomplish what you needed to accomplish.

The ending should consume about 20 percent of the time. It should focus on the results, the cost savings, bonuses, awards, and promotions (the outcome) that came about because of your action in the situation.

FOCUS ON THE POSITIVE

It is critical that you accentuate the positive in your story. Negative comments and emotions create negative impressions. Likewise, the inability to manage the story and the time you spend responding creates a negative impression as well.

Make sure you come across as positive by doing or not doing the following:

1. Don't whine. A whiny story leads the interviewer to assume you will whine as a student as well.
2. Do not bad-mouth anyone. Someone who bad-mouths others in an interview story is likely to do that as a student as well.

3. Keep your answers to three minutes. *Short* and *succinct* are words to remember as you respond to the question.
4.   Don't ramble about irrelevant details. Get to the point and keep to the point.
5. Watch your language. Don't use inappropriate language or slang. Make sure you use language that best represents who you are as a person.

COMMON PROBLEMS ENCOUNTERED IN ANSWERING SITUATIONAL QUESTIONS

*   Spending too much time setting up the story
*   Not providing enough information in the middle of the story—The interviewee simplifies the action, making it sound like an easy task or problem when it was actually very difficult and involved a great deal of effort above and beyond the norm.
*   Not having an ending to the story—What was the outcome? The interviewer is left wondering, *What happened next?*

SAMPLE QUESTIONS

As I mentioned earlier, situational interview questions are designed to test your judgment and your analytical and problem-solving skills. The following is a list of common PA school situational interview questions and answers.

Q: During a clinical rotation as a PA school student, one of your chief medical residents has a thick accent and you have difficulty understanding him on rounds. What would you do?

A: This is a difficult situation, as I do not think I would actually confront the resident myself. I would make every effort to actively listen and do my best to understand what he is saying. I would also ask a lot of questions to clarify anything that is unclear to me, and I would compare notes with my fellow students after rounds were over. This way, I could make sure that I understood what he said. Discussing it afterward would help reinforce the things I learned during rounds.

Q: List the steps you would take to make an acute decision relative to a patient's care in the intensive care unit.

A: My steps would include asking the following questions:

1. Would my decision cause harm to the patient?
2. Do I need to make this decision now?
3. Do I need to consult my supervising physician?

Q: You are a PA on the hospitalist service in a large hospital. One of the hospital residents writes an order for IV potassium in the patient's chart, and you disagree with that order. What would you do?

A: I would first make a case for why the patient does not need the potassium and then consider the harmful effects that could follow if the patient did in fact receive it. Then I would call/page the resident and express my concerns. If the resident did not agree, I would tell the resident that I do not feel comfortable ordering this medication and I would document our conversation in the patient's chart. I would *not* order the medication if I knew it was going to harm the patient.

Q: You witness a colleague (Joe) stealing controlled medications from the drug cabinet. When confronted, he tells you that they are for a friend who has no health insurance and cannot afford the medication. What do you do?

A: I would confront Joe and say, "Joe, I witnessed you taking controlled medications and putting them into your pocket. I am very concerned that you are jeopardizing your medical license and mine. I am not willing to stand by and do nothing. If you don't return the medication, I am going to have to report you to the appropriate authorities. If you put them back now, we can sit down and figure out a solution that does not involve jeopardizing your career. Otherwise, I am obliged to report this incident."

Q: You are the first assistant in the operating room for a cardiothoracic surgery case. While scrubbing in for the procedure, you notice that the cardiac surgeon, also scrubbing next to you, has the smell of alcohol on his breath. What do you do?

A: I would say, "Dr. Smith, your breath smells like alcohol to me. I am concerned that you may be impaired. If you have been drinking, I cannot participate in this case, and I will have to notify the anesthesiologist and the scrub nurses participating in this procedure. If you reschedule the case or find another surgeon to perform the procedure, I will not have to report you."

Q: You are a first-year PA student, and you witness one of your classmates cheating on her examination. What would you do?

A: I would confront the student after the examination and tell her that I saw her referring to an index card in her coat pocket and then penciling in the answers to the test questions. I would tell her that I feel uncomfortable with this situation and I cannot let it continue. I would then ask her what she thinks we ought to do about it. In any case, I would not allow her to continue cheating on exams.

Q: You are on a clinical rotation in OB-GYN, and your attending physician often leaves you alone and asks you to do things that are outside the scope of practice for a PA student. You really like the rotation and the attending physician, but you are concerned that you may be crossing the boundaries between a student and a licensed practitioner. What would you do?

A: I would have a discussion with the attending physician and, first, tell him how much I appreciate the confidence he has shown in me. I would then describe exactly what I have been doing that is out of the scope of my practice as a PA student. I would tell him that I feel liable for some of the decisions I am making and that, as a student, I am not willing to accept that liability. I would offer to share the PA program's description of responsibilities and duties while on clinical rotations and tell him that I am perfectly willing to participate in any of these activities.

Q: After working a "double" shift, you realize that you gave a patient the wrong medication. The patient seems to be doing fine, but you are concerned. What do you do?

A: The first rule of medicine is to "do no harm." I would double-check the medication to see if what I prescribed would be harmful to the patient or interact with any of her prescribed medications. I would then check the patient's vital signs and look for any suggestion of an adverse reaction. I would speak to the patient directly, informing her that I made a medication error and that she appears to be stable. I would ask her if she had any questions or concerns relative to the medication error. I would then document the facts surrounding the error in the patient's chart and order the correct medication. I would also notify my supervisor about the incident.

Q: You work in a well-known dermatology practice where you are used to having a great deal of autonomy. One day, your supervising physician calls you into her office to tell you that she invested in a new laser system for weight loss, and she would like you to perform the procedures. She also informs you that she will be working in a satellite office three days a week, and you will be alone on those days. You check the state laws regarding physician assistants and laser procedures and learn that you must have your supervising physician on the premises at all times when using the laser. When you relay this information to the dermatologist, she says, "Don't worry about it, there are no laser police!" What do you do?

A: I would tell the dermatologist that I am extremely excited about training on the new laser and that I appreciate her confidence in me. Although I am very comfortable working autonomously, I feel like I am risking my medical license if I don't abide by the state laws governing PAs and laser treatments. I am just not willing to risk my license to practice medicine. However, if we can find a way to book the procedures on the days that she is there in that office, I would be more than happy to perform the treatments.

Q: You are working on the orthopedic floor of a large hospital when the entire staff is briefed about an impending medical malpractice suit from a former patient. Later that day, you notice one of your colleagues pulled the patient's chart and is altering some of his notes. What do you do?

A: I would speak to my colleague, in private, and tell him that I saw him making alterations in the chart of the person who may be filing the lawsuit. I would tell him that I am concerned that he may be trying to cover up a mistake and if that were the case, I would not cover for him if he gets caught. I would tell him if he notifies staff that he made changes to the chart, he may be able to avoid legal action and losing his medical license. If he did not cooperate, I would have no choice but to notify our superiors myself.

Illegal questions

7

Similar to writing good test questions, selecting appropriate interview questions is a skill. Most PA school admissions committee members are not professional interviewers and may not even know what constitutes an "illegal" question. Questions should be related to your qualifications to become a PA, not to personal information about you.

When dealing with illegal questions, you have to ask yourself: Do I want to be "right" or effective?

Here's the dilemma: if you are asked an illegal question, do you respond, "Hey, that's an illegal question"?

Even if you knew, absolutely, that the interviewers knew what they are doing, you might be tempted to become upset. But what if the interviewers are asking the question out of ignorance? Would you look at the situation from a different perspective?

For the purpose of being effective, versus being "right," I recommend that you assume the interviewers asked the illegal question out of ignorance. However, you don't have to answer the question directly. In this chapter, I will provide you with a list of illegal questions/topics and make some recommendations as to how you can respond.

Which questions are illegal?

Questions about marital/family status:

"Do you have any children?"

The interviewer may ask you this question to determine in his mind ("fortune-telling") if you will need to take time off from school or rotations to stay home with your children.

The best way to answer is: "There is nothing in my family situation that will interfere with my ability to attend class or clinical rotations."

Similar questions to consider:

"Are you married?"

"Are you planning to have children?"

"Are you pregnant?"

"Who is going to watch your children when you're in school?"

Questions about age

"How old are you?"

This question probably has more to do with maturity than chronological age.

The best way to answer is: "I've accomplished all of the academic prerequisites and medical experience requirements to qualify for this program. I know what it takes to become a good physician assistant, and I am ready to embrace the challenges of PA school."

Similar questions to consider:

"When were you born?"

"When is your birthday?"

Personal questions

"How much do you weigh?"

This is a rude and illegal question to say the least. The interviewer may be thinking that you cannot handle the job if you are overweight or obese. The interviewer may also be extremely judgmental.

The best way to answer is: "Weight has never been an issue for me. I've never had a problem performing any of my job duties."

Similar questions to consider:

"How tall are you?"

"What is your sexual orientation?"

Questions about disabilities

"I see you're not moving your arm; did you hurt yourself?"

This is a "fishing" question to see if you have a disability that would interfere with your duties as a PA.

The best way to answer is: "I'm fine, thank you." That's it, no need to elaborate.

Similar questions to consider:

"What medications do you take?"

"Do you have any mental health issues?"

"Do you have heart disease?"

"Have you ever been treated for alcoholism or drug addiction?"

"Do you have an eating disorder?"

"Will you need us to make any accommodations in order for you to complete the program?"

Questions about national origin / citizenship

"You have an interesting accent; which country are you from?"

Inquiries about a person's citizenship or country of birth are unlawful and imply discrimination on the basis of national origin.

The best way to answer is: "That's an interesting question. Is that information pertinent to my application?"

Similar questions to consider:

"Where were you born?"

"Are you a citizen?"

"Your last name sounds Italian, is it?"

Questions about your arrest record

"Have you ever been arrested?"

Upon completion of PA school, you will have to undergo a background check to see if you qualify for a medical license. If you have any felonies or drug convictions, you will be disqualified. You may want to check this out for yourself before applying.

However, if you have been arrested for any minor offenses but not convicted, you don't have to divulge that information. If you have a current arrest, the admissions committee can ask you about that and take it into consideration when making a decision about your candidacy.

The best way to answer is: "No. I've never been convicted of a criminal offense."

Similar questions to consider:

"Have you ever committed a crime?"

Questions about military service

"Have you ever served in the military, or are you currently on active duty?"

Even though the PA profession got its start with former U.S. Navy corpsman, don't assume that all of the admissions committee members are pro-military.

If your military training is relevant and supportive of your application to PA school, you may want to elaborate on the specifics of your training and job. However, be cautious about your answers and about divulging too much information.

The best way to answer is: "Yes, I received an honorable discharge from the navy in 1999."

Questions about politics/affiliations

"Are you a Republican or a Democrat?"

This is a loaded question. Never talk about politics at an interview, unless you want to sabotage your chances of being accepted.

The best way to answer is: "It is my policy never to discuss politics with anyone."

Similar questions to consider:

"Who did you vote for in the last election?"

"Are you in a union?"

"What do you think about the president?"

Questions about race / color / religion

All questions about these topics are illegal. Interviewers may ask about your religious background to see if you will have any conflict working Saturdays or Sundays.

The best way to answer is: "My religious preference is very personal."

"Are you Caucasian / African American / Hispanic?"

"Do you attend church/ synagogue / mosque?"

After the Interview and Final Thoughts

8

AFTER THE INTERVIEW

The interview is over, and you have done your best. Now you can just sit back and wait, right? Wrong. There a few dos and don'ts for after the interview.

Do follow up with a written thank-you note within two business days of the interview. Make sure to use professional (not flowery) stationary. In that note, thank them for their time and offer to discuss with them any additional information they might need.

Don't follow up with an e-mail thank-you. Interviewers get too many e-mails as it is, and you don't want to contribute to their inbox overflow. Additionally, e-mail thank-yous are easy and imply that you didn't want to take the time to send a hand-written thank-you.

Do use the correct titles and names for all of those who interviewed you so you can get thank-you notes correct. If possible, get business cards during the interview.

Do use the thank-you letter as an opportunity to continue to advance yourself as a candidate and also to show your fit with the school. Now that you have more specifics on the program, you can make a comment or two (no more—remember, this is primarily a thank-you note) about how you fit well with the program and why you will be a good student.

Don't make a pest of yourself. Follow up is good, but you don't want to communicate so much that your communication becomes a burden for your potential program.

FINAL THOUGHTS.

Remember, prepare for your PA school interview like you would for a job interview with a corporation. Learn everything there is to know about that school so you can show them why you would be a good fit for that program and why they should select you over another applicant. To do this, you must be relaxed and conversational, make good eye contact, and anticipate which questions you'll be asked during the interview at each specific program.

Remember that "communication is a contact sport." Use eye contact, open gestures, and variety in your tone of voice to create trust. If you speak in a monotone and avoid eye contact with everyone involved in the interview, you're likely to isolate some members and not achieve a high score.

Remember to sell yourself:

- Grab the attention of the interviewer.
- Create an interest by telling stories and vignettes.
- Demonstrate conviction by pointing out your hard work to get there.
- Create a desire to have you as a member of the incoming class by using "high-impact" communication skills.
- Close the deal with a relaxed, confident posture.

Remember, if you are a strong applicant, the program will want you as much as you want them. Don't sell yourself short. The trick is to ask questions to maintain a certain control that lets the committee know you are checking out their program as much as they are checking you out. If you are a strong applicant, you can pull this off effectively.

Remember to practice, practice, and practice some more.

Interviewing is a learned skill that takes lots of practice. The first thing you need to do is anticipate the questions that you will be asked and formulate your answers. Remember, for behavioral questions, you must tell a story! Use the templates above or anything that works for you.

Most important, *remember, failure to prepare is preparing to fail!*

Resources for PA School Applicants

9

AJR ASSOCIATES

AJR Associates (www.Andrew Rodican.com) was founded in 1997 by the author, Andrew J. Rodican, PA-C. His company is solely dedicated to helping PA school applicants achieve success. Some of the services Mr. Rodican offers include:

- Application review, assessment, and recommendations
- Essay review and edit
- "Mock: interviews via Skype
- Unlimited email support
- Seminars on DVD
- Workbooks

Please visit www.AndrewRodican,com for more information, or contact Mr. Rodican directly at AJR@AndrewRodican.com.

AMERICAN ACADEMY OF PHYSICIAN ASSISTANTS (AAPA)

The American Academy of Physician Assistants (AAPA) is the only national professional association that represents all PAs across all medical and surgical specialties in all 50 states, the District of Columbia, Guam, the armed forces, and the federal services.

AAPA provides comprehensive support and advocacy for physician assistants so that they may, in turn, provide patients with increased access to quality, cost-effective health care.

HISTORY

Founded in 1968 to support the growing PA profession, AAPA works to increase the professional and personal growth of the more than 73,000 PAs in practice today through a range of information, advocacy and services.

MEMBERS

Physician assistants who are graduates of PA educational programs accredited by the Accreditation Review Commission on Education for the Physician Assistant (ARC-PA) or one of its predecessor agencies are eligible for fellow membership member in AAPA. There are other membership categories for PA students, physicians, PAs who are no longer practicing but wish to support the profession, other health professionals, and service providers.

CONTACT

American Academy of Physician Assistants
2318 Mill Road, Suite 1300
Alexandria, VA 22314
p. 703.836.2272 f. 703.684.1924
aapa@aapa.org

STUDENT ACADEMY OF THE AMERICAN ACADEMY OF PHYSICIAN ASSISTANTS (SAAAPA)

The Student Academy of the American Academy of Physician Assistants is **dedicated to PA students** and provides them with useful and current information related to being a PA student and the PA profession.

The SAAAPA is a great resource for PA school applicants who would like to contact student PAs from various PA programs around the country.

CONTACT

http://aapa.org/student-academy

PA FORUM

Established in 1998, the physician assistant forum has become the largest online social network of physician assistants, physician assistant students and those interested in becoming a physician assistant. The forum has over 13 years of experience related information and physician assistant jobs or employment opportunities. The forum also has a large physician assistant school section with tons of helpful information for applying and interviews.

PA School applicants are invited to register and post comments on the forum.

CONTACT

http://www.physicianassistantforum.com/forums/forum.php

PHYSICIAN ASSISTANT EDUCATION ASSOCIATION (PAEA)

The Physician Assistant Education Association (PAEA) is the only national organization in the United States representing physician assistant (PA) educational programs. PAEA serves as a resource for individuals and organizations from various professional sectors interested in the educational aspects of the PA profession. The Association is the organization primarily responsible for collecting, publishing, and disseminating information on the PA programs. PAEA provides effective representation to affiliated organizations involved in health education, health care policy, and the national certification of PA graduates. PAEA works to ensure quality PA education through the development and distribution of educational services and products specifically geared toward meeting the emerging needs of PA programs, the PA profession, and the health care industry.

CONTACT

http://www.paeaonline.org/index.php?ht=d/sp/i/212/pid/212

NATIONAL COMMISSION ON CERTIFICATION OF PHYSICIAN ASSISTANTS (NCCPA)

NCCPA is the only credentialing organization for physician assistants in the United States. Established as a not-for-profit organization in 1975, NCCPA is dedicated to assuring the public that certified physician assistants meet established standards of knowledge and clinical skills upon entry into practice and throughout their careers. Every U.S. state, the District of Columbia and the U.S. territories have decided to rely on NCCPA certification as one of the criteria for licensure or regulation of physician assistants. Approximately 86,000 physician assistants have been certified by NCCPA.

CONTACT

http://www.nccpa.net/

ACCREDITATION REVIEW COMMISSION ON EDUCATION FOR THE PHYSICIAN ASSISTANT (ARC-PA)

The Accreditation Review Commission on Education for the Physician Assistant is the accrediting agency that protects the interests of the public and physician assistant profession by defining the standards for physician assistant education and evaluating physician assistant educational programs within the territorial United States to ensure their compliance with those standards.
http://www.arc-pa.org/

AAPA CONSTITUENT CHAPTERS

Society of Air Force Physician Assistants
http://www.safpa.org/
Alabama Society of Physician Assistants
http://www.myaspa.org/
Alaska Academy of Physician Assistants
http://www.akapa.org/
Arizona State Association of Physician Assistants
http://www.asapa.org/
Arkansas Academy of Physician Assistants
http://www.arkansaspa.org/
Society of Army Physician Assistants
http://www.sapa.org/
California Academy of Physician Assistants
http://www.capanet.org/
Colorado Academy of Physician Assistants
http://www.coloradopas.org/
Connecticut Academy of Physician Assistants
http://www.connapa.org/
Delaware Academy of Physician Assistants
http://www.delawarepas.org
District of Columbia Academy of Physician Assistants
http://www.dcapa.org/
Florida Academy of Physician Assistants
http://www.fapaonline.org/
Georgia Association of Physician Assistants
http://www.gapa.net/
Hawaii Academy of Physician Assistants
http://www.hapahawaii.org/
Idaho Academy of Physician Assistants
http://www.idahopa.org/
Illinois Academy of Physician Assistants
http://www.illinoispa.org/
Indiana Academy of Physician Assistants
http://www.indianapas.org/

Iowa Physician Assistant Society
http://www.iapasociety.org/
Kansas Academy of Physician Assistants
http://www.kansaspa.com/
Kentucky Academy of Physician Assistants
http://www.kentuckypa.org/
Louisiana Academy of Physician Assistants
http://www.ourlapa.org/
Downeast Association of PAs
http://www.deapa.com/
Maryland Academy of Physician Assistants
http://www.mdapa.org/menumain.asp
Massachusetts Association of Physician Assistants
http://www.mass-pa.com/
Michigan Academy of Physician Assistants
http://www.michiganpa.org/AM/Template.cfm?Section=Home2
Minnesota Academy of Physician Assistants
http://www.mnacadpa.org/
Mississippi Academy of Physician Assistants
http://www.missipas.org/
Missouri Academy of Physician Assistants
http://www.moapa.org/
Montana Academy of Physician Assistants
http://www.mtapa.com/
Naval Association of Physician Assistants
http://www.napasite.net/
Nebraska Academy of Physician Assistants
http://www.nebraskapa.org/
Nevada Academy of Physician Assistants
http://www.nevadapa.com/
New Hampshire Society of Physician Assistants
http://www.nh-spa.org/
New Jersey State Society of Physician Assistants
http://www.njsspa.org/
New Mexico Academy of Physician Assistants
http://www.nmapa.com/
New York State Society of Physician Assistants

http://www.nysspa.org/
North Carolina Academy of Physician Assistants
http://www.ncapa.org/
North Dakota Academy of Physician Assistants
http://www.ndapahome.org/
Ohio Association of Physician Assistants
http://www.ohiopa.com/
Oklahoma Academy of Physician Assistants
http://www.okpa.org/
Oregon Society of Physician Assistants
http://www.oregonpa.org/
Pennsylvania Society of PAs
http://www.pspa.net/index.html
Public Health Service Academy of Physician Assistants
http://phsapa.com
Rhode Island Academy of Physician Assistants
http://www.myriapa.org/
South Carolina Academy of Physician Assistants
http://www.scapapartners.org/
South Dakota Academy of Physician Assistants
http://www.sdapa.net/
Tennessee Academy of Physician Assistants
http://www.tnpa.com/
Texas Academy of Physician Assistants
http://www.tapa.org/
Utah Academy of Physician Assistants
http://www.utahapa.org/
Physician Assistant Academy of Vermont
http://www.paav.org/
Veterans Affairs Physician Assistant Association
http://www.vapaa.org/
Virginia Academy of Physician Assistants
http://www.vapa.org/
Washington State Academy of Physician Assistants
http://www.wapa.com/
West Virginia Association of Physician Assistants
http://www.mywvapa.org/

Wisconsin Academy of Physician Assistants
http://www.wapa.org/
Wyoming Association of Physician Assistants
http://www.wapa.net/

U.S. PA PROGRAMS ACCREDITED BY ARC-PA
ALABAMA

University of Alabama at Birmingham
Surgical Physician Assistant Program
School of Health Related Professions
RMSB 481; 1530 3rd Avenue South
Birmingham, AL
35294-1212
Phone: (205) 934-4605
http://main.uab.edu/Shrp/Default.aspx?pid=32650
University of South Alabama
Department of Physician Assistant Studies
1504 Springhill Avenue, Suite 4410
Mobile, AL
36604-3273
Phone: (251) 434-3641
http://www.southalabama.edu/alliedhealth/pa/

ARIZONA

Arizona School of Health Sciences
Physician Assistant Program
5850 East Still Circle
Mesa, AZ
85206
Phone: (480) 219-6000
http://www.atsu.edu/ashs/programs/physician_assistant/napa.htm
Midwestern University
Office of Admissions

Physician Assistant Program
19555 North 59th Avenue
Glendale, AZ
85308-6813
http://www.midwestern.edu/Programs_and_Admission/
AZ_Physician_Assistant_Studies.html

ARKANSAS

Harding University
Physician Assistant Program
Box 12231
Searcy, AR
72149
Phone: (501) 279-5642
http://www.harding.edu/PAprogram/

ARMED FORCES

Interservice Physician Assistant Program
Academy of Health Sciences
Attn: MCCSHMP
3151 Scott Road, Suite 1302
Fort Sam Houston,TX, UN
78234-6138
Phone: (210) 221-8004
http://www.usarec.army.mil/armypa/

CALIFORNIA

Charles R. Drew University of Medicine and Science
Physician Assistant Program
College of Health Sciences

1731 East 120th Street
Los Angeles, CA
90059
Phone: (323) 563-5879
http://www.allalliedhealthschools.com/find/show.php?id=1672

KECK SCHOOL OF MEDICINE OF THE UNIVERSITY OF SOUTHERN

California
Physician Assistant Program
Department of Family Medicine
1000 South Fremont Avenue, Unit 7, Bldg. A-6, Rm. 6429
Alhambra, CA
91803-8897
Phone: (626) 457-4240
http://www.usc.edu/schools/medicine/departments/
physician_assistant/

LOMA LINDA UNIVERSITY

Physician Assistant Program
School of Allied Health Professions
Nichol Hall, Room 2033
Loma Linda, CA
92350
Phone: (909) 558-7295
http://www.llu.edu/llu/sahp/pa/

RIVERSIDE COUNTY REGIONAL MEDICAL CENTER/ RIVERSIDE

Community College
Primary Care PA Program

16130 Lasselle Street
Moreno Valley, CA
92551
Phone: (951) 571-6166
http://www.rcc.edu/academicPrograms/physicianAssistant/

SAMUEL MERRITT UNIVERSITY

Physician Assistant Program
450 30th Street, Ste. 4708
Oakland, CA
94609
Phone: (510) 869-6623
http://www.samuelmerritt.edu/physician_assistant

SAN JOAQUIN VALLEY COLLEGE

Primary Care PA Program
8400 West Mineral King Avenue
Visalia, CA
93291
Phone: (559) 651-2500 ext. 351
http://www.sjvc.edu/programs/programs.php?programID=26

STANFORD UNIVERSITY SCHOOL OF MEDICINE

Primary Care Associate Program
Family Nurse Practitioner
Physician Assistant Program
1215 Welch Road, Modular G
Palo Alto, CA
94305-5408
Phone: (650) 725-6959
http://pcap.stanford.edu/program/pa.html

TOURO UNIVERSITY—CALIFORNIA COLLEGE OF HEALTH SCIENCES

Physician Assistant Program
Office of Admissions
1310 Johnson Lane
Vallejo, CA
94592
Phone: (888) 652-7580
http://www.tu.edu/departments.php?id=50&page=610

UNIVERSITY OF CALIFORNIA—DAVIS

Physician Assistant Program
Family Nurse Practitioner Program
Department of Family and Community Medicine
2516 Stockton Blvd, Suite 254
Sacramento, CA
95817-2208
Phone: (916) 734-3551
http://www.ucdmc.ucdavis.edu/fnppa/

WESTERN UNIVERSITY OF HEALTH SCIENCES

Primary Care Physician Assistant Program
309 E. Second Street
Pomona, CA
91766-1854
Phone: (909) 469-5378
http://www.westernu.edu/xp/edu/cahp/mspas_about.xml

COLORADO

Red Rocks Community College
Physician Assistant Program
13300 West 6th Avenue
Denver, CO
80228-1255
Phone: (303) 914-6386
http://www.rrcc.edu/pa/
University of Colorado at Denver and Health Sciences Center
Child Health Associate
Physician Assistant Program
PO Box 6508, Mail Stop F543
Aurora, CO
80045
Phone: (303) 315-7963
http://www.uchsc.edu/chapa/

CONNECTICUT

Quinnipiac University
Physician Assistant Program
Office of Graduate Admissions (AB-GRD)
275 Mount Carmel Avenue
Hamden, CT
06518-1908
Phone: (203) 582-8672
http://www.quinnipiac.edu/x781.xml

YALE UNIVERSITY SCHOOL OF MEDICINE

Physician Associate Program
367 Cedar Street

Harkness Office Building, 2nd Floor
New Haven, CT
06510
Phone: (203) 785-2860
http://medicine.yale.edu/pa/

WASHINGTON, D.C.

George Washington University
Physician Assistant Program
900 23rd Street NW , Suite 6148
Washington, DC
20037
Phone: (202) 994-6661
http://www.gwumc.edu/healthsci/programs/pa/

HOWARD UNIVERSITY

Physician Assistant Program
College of Pharmacy, Nursing and Allied Health Sciences
6th & Bryant Street, NW , Annex I
Washington, DC
20059
Phone: (202) 806-7536
http://www.cpnahs.howard.edu/AHS/Pa/Introduction.htm

FLORIDA

Barry University School of Graduate Medical Sciences
Physician Assistant Program
11300 NE Second Avenue, Box SGMS
Miami Shores, FL
33161

Phone: (305) 899-3296

http://www.barry.edu/pa/

MIAMI DADE COLLEGE

Physician Assistant Program

Medical Center Campus

950 NW 20th Street

Miami, FL

33127-4693

Phone: (305) 237-4124

http://www.mdc.edu/medical/academic_programs/
physician_assistant/physician.htm

NOVA SOUTHEASTERN UNIVERSITY, FT. LAUDERDALE

Physician Assistant Program

3200 South University Dr.

Fort Lauderdale, FL

33328

Phone: (954) 262-1250

http://www.nova.edu/pa/

NOVA SOUTHEASTERN UNIVERSITY, JACKSONVILLE

Physician Assistant Program

6675 Corporate Center Parkway, Suite 112

Jacksonville, FL

32216

Phone: (904) 245-8990

http://www.nova.edu/pa/jacksonville/

NOVA SOUTHEASTERN UNIVERSITY, ORLANDO

Physician Assistant Program
4850 Millenia Boulevard
Orlando, FL
32839
Phone: (407) 264-5150
http://www.nova.edu/pa/orlando/

NOVA SOUTHEASTERN UNIVERSITY, SOUTHWEST FLORIDA

Physician Assistant Program
2655 Northbrooke Drive
Naples, FL
34119
Phone: (239) 591-4528 ext. 20
http://www.nova.edu/pa/swflorida/

UNIVERSITY OF FLORIDA

Physician Assistant Program
PO Box 100176
Gainesville, FL
32610-0176
Phone: (352) 265-7955
http://www.med.ufl.edu/pap/apply/

GEORGIA

Emory University School of Medicine
Physician Assistant Program
Department of Family and Preventive Medicine
1462 Clifton Rd, Suite 280

Atlanta, GA
30322
Phone: (404) 727-7825
http://www.emorypa.org/

MEDICAL COLLEGE OF GEORGIA

Physician Assistant Program
Physician Assistant Department
EC-3304
Augusta, GA
30912
Phone: (706) 721-3246
http://www.mcg.edu/students/semcon/corefpa.htm

MERCER UNIVERSITY COLLEGE OF PHARMACY AND HEALTH SCIENCES

Physician Assistant Program
3001 Mercer University Drive
Atlanta, GA
30341
Phone: (678-547-6214
http://cophs.mercer.edu/pa.htm

SOUTH UNIVERSITY

Physician Assistant Program
709 Mall Blvd.
Savannah, GA
31406
Phone: (912) 201-8025
http://www.southuniversity.edu/PhysicianAssistant/

IDAHO

Idaho State University
Department of Physician Assistant Studies
Campus Box 8253
1021 S Red Hill Road
Pocatello, ID
83209-8253
Phone: (208) 282-4726
http://www.isu.edu/PAprog/

IOWA

Des Moines University
Physician Assistant Program
3200 Grand Avenue
Des Moines, IA
50312
Phone: (515) 271-7854
http://www.dmu.edu/chs/pa/
University of Iowa
Physician Assistant Program
Carver College of Medicine
5167 Westlawn
Iowa City, IA
52242-1100
Phone: (319) 335-8922
http://paprogram.medicine.uiowa.edu/

ILLINOIS

**John H. Stroger Jr. Hospital of Cook County/
Malcolm X College**
Physician Assistant Program
1900 W. Van Buren, #3241

Chicago, IL
60612
Phone: (312) 850-7255
http://malcolmx.ccc.edu/Academic_Programs/

PHYSICIANASSISTANT.ASP

Midwestern University
Physician Assistant Program
555 31st Street
Downers Grove, IL
60515
Phone: (800) 458-6253
http://www.midwestern.edu/Programs_and_Admission/
IL_Physician_Assistant_Studies.html

ROSALIND FRANKLIN UNIVERSITY OF MEDICINE AND SCIENCE

Physician Assistant Program
3333 Green Bay Road
North Chicago, IL
60064-3095
Phone: (847) 589-8686
http://www.rosalindfranklin.edu/DNN/home/CHP/PA/MS/
tabid/1570/Default.aspx

SOUTHERN ILLINOIS UNIVERSITY AT CARBONDALE

Physician Assistant Program
Lindegren Hall, Room 129, Mail Code 6516
Carbondale, IL
62901-6516
Phone: (618) 453-5527
http://www.siu.edu/~sah/pa.html

INDIANA

Butler University/Clarian Health
Physician Assistant Program
College of Pharmacy and Health Sciences
4600 Sunset Avenue
Indianapolis, IN
46208
Phone: (317) 940-9969
http://www.butler.edu/cophs/?pg=2077&parentID=2041

UNIVERSITY OF SAINT FRANCIS

Physician Assistant Program
2701 Spring Street
Fort Wayne, IN
46808
Phone: (260) 434-7737
http://www.sf.edu/healthscience/pa/msentryprogram.shtml

KANSAS

Wichita State University
Physician Assistant Program
College of Health Professions
1845 N. Fairmount, Box 43
Wichita, KS
67260-0043
Phone: (316) 978-3011
http://webs.wichita.edu/?u=chp_pa&p=/index

KENTUCKY

University of Kentucky
Physician Assistant Program

College of Health Sciences
900 S. Limestone Street, Suite 205
Lexington, KY
40536-0200
Phone: (859) 323-1100
http://www.mc.uky.edu/PA/

LOUISIANA

Louisiana State University Health Sciences Center
Physician Assistant Program
School of Allied Health Professions
1501 Kings Highway, PO Box 33932
Shreveport, LA
71130-3932
Phone: (318) 675-7317
http://www.universities.com/edu/Louisiana_State_University__
Health_Sciences_Center_Bachelor_degree_Physician_Assistant.html

OUR LADY OF THE LAKE COLLEGE

Physician Associate Program
7443 Picardy Avenue
Baton Rouge, LA
70808
Phone: (225) 214-6988
http://www.ololcollege.edu/physician_asst.html

MASSACHUSETTS

Massachusetts College of Pharmacy and Health Sciences
Physician Assistant Studies Program
179 Longwood Avenue, W110
Boston, MA

02115
Phone: (617) 732-2918
http://www.mcphs.edu/academics/programs/physician_assistant_
studies/

NORTHEASTERN UNIVERSITY

Physician Assistant Program
360 Huntington Ave
202 Robinson Hall
Boston, MA
02115
Phone: (617) 373-3195
http://www.northeastern.edu/bouve/programs/mphysassist/
mphysassist.html

SPRINGFIELD COLLEGE/BAYSTATE HEALTH SYSTEM

Physician Assistant Program
263 Alden Street
Springfield, MA
01109
Phone: (800) 343-1257
http://catalog.spfldcol.edu/preview_program.php?catoid=26&poid=
891&bc=1

MARYLAND

Anne Arundel Community College
Physician Assistant Program
School of Health Professions, Wellness and Physical Education
101 College Parkway

Arnold, MD
21012
Phone: (410) 777-7310
http://www.aacc.edu/physassist/Admissions.cfm

TOWSON UNIVERSITY, CCBC ESSEX

Physician Assistant Program
7201 Rossville Boulevard
Baltimore, MD
21237-1899
Phone: (410) 780-6159
http://www.towson.edu/chp/pa/

UNIVERSITY OF MARYLAND, EASTERN SHORE

Physician Assistant Program
Haze Hall, Room 1034
Princess Anne, MD
21853
Phone: (410) 651-7584
http://www.umes.edu/PA/Default.aspx?id=2408

MAINE

University of New England
Physician Assistant Program
716 Stevens Avenue
Biddeford, ME
04103-7688
Phone: (207) 221-4529
http://www.une.edu/chp/pa/

MICHIGAN

Central Michigan University
Physician Assistant Program
1222 Health Professions Bldg
Mount Pleasant, MI
48859
Phone: (989) 774-2478
http://www.gradschools.com/Program/MI_United-States/
Graduate-Program-Physician-Assistant/205187.html

GRAND VALLEY STATE UNIVERSITY

Physician Assistant Program
301 Michigan Street, NE, Ste. 200 CHS
Grand Rapids, MI
49503
Phone: (616) 331-3356
http://www.gvsu.edu/pas/

UNIVERSITY OF DETROIT MERCY

Physician Assistant Program
4001 West McNichols Road
Detroit, MI
48221
Phone: (313) 993-2474
http://www.udmercy.edu/apply/financial_aid/type/
health-professions/physician-assistant/index.htm

WAYNE STATE UNIVERSITY

Department of Physician Assistant Studies
259 Mack Avenue, Ste. 2590

Detroit, MI
48201
Phone: (313) 577-1368
http://www.pa.cphs.wayne.edu/

WESTERN MICHIGAN UNIVERSITY

Physician Assistant Program
1903 West Michigan Avenue
Kalamazoo, MI
49008-5138
Phone: (269) 387-5314
http://www.wmich.edu/paprog/

MINNESOTA

Augsburg College
Physician Assistant Program
Campus Box 149
2211 Riverside Avenue
Minneapolis, MN
55454
Phone: (612) 330-1399
http://www.augsburg.edu/pa/

MISSOURI

Missouri State University
Department of Physician Assistant Studies
901 S. National PTPA 112
Springfield, MO
65897
Phone: (417) 836-6151
http://www.missouristate.edu/pas/

SAINT LOUIS UNIVERSITY

Physician Assistant Program
Doisy College of Health Sciences
3437 Caroline Street
St. Louis, MO
63104-1111
Phone: (314) 977-8521
http://www.slu.edu/x2348.xml

MONTANA

Rocky Mountain College—M
Physician Assistant Program
1511 Poly Drive
Billings, MT
59102-1739
Phone: (406) 657-1190
http://www.rocky.edu/academics/programs/mpas/Admissions.shtml

NORTH CAROLINA

Duke University Medical Center
Physician Assistant Program
DUMC 3848
Durham, NC
27710
Phone: (919) 681-3161
http://paprogram.mc.duke.edu/

EAST CAROLINA UNIVERSITY

Physician Assistant Program
School of Allied Health Sciences

Health Sciences Building, Suite 4310
Greenville, NC
27858-4353
Phone: (252) 744-1100
http://www.ecu.edu/pa/

METHODIST UNIVERSITY

Physician Assistant Program
5107B College Centre Drive
Fayetteville, NC
28311
Phone: (910) 630-7495
http://www.methodist.edu/paprogram/

WAKE FOREST UNIVERSITY

Physician Assistant Program
Medical Center Boulevard
Winston-Salem, NC
27157-1006
Phone: (336) 716-4356
http://www1.wfubmc.edu/PAprogram/

WINGATE UNIVERSITY

Physician Assistant Program
Campus Box 5010
Wingate, NC
28174
Phone: (704) 233-8051
http://pa.wingate.edu/

NORTH DAKOTA

University of North Dakota School of Medicine and Health
Sciences
Physician Assistant Program
Department of Family and Community Medicine
501 N. Columbia Road—Stop 9037, Room 4128
Grand Forks, ND
58202-9037
Phone: (701) 777-2344
http://www.med.und.nodak.edu/physicianassistant/

NEBRASKA

Union College
Physician Assistant Program
3800 South 48th Street
Lincoln, NE
68506
Phone: (402) 486-2527
http://www.ucollege.edu/?DivID=1&pgID=301

UNIVERSITY OF NEBRASKA MEDICAL CENTER

Physician Assistant Program
984300 Nebraska Medical Center
Omaha, NE
68198-4300
Phone: (402) 559-9495
http://www.unmc.edu/alliedhealth/pa/

NEW HAMPSHIRE

Massachusetts College of Pharmacy and Health Sciences,
Manchester

PA Program
1260 Elm Street
Manchester, NH
03101
Phone: (603) 314-1730
http://www.mcphs.edu/academics/programs/
physician_assistant_studies/PA_24_Man/

NEW JERSEY

Seton Hall University
Physician Assistant Program
400 South Orange Avenue
South Orange, NJ
07079-2689
Phone: (973) 275-2596
http://www.shu.edu/academics/gradmeded/
ms-physician-assistant/index.cfm

UNIVERSITY OF MEDICINE AND DENTISTRY OF NEW JERSEY

Physician Assistant Program
Robert Wood Johnson Medical School
675 Hoes Lane
Piscataway, NJ
08854-5635
Phone: (732) 235-4445
http://shrp.umdnj.edu/programs/paweb/

NEW MEXICO

University of New Mexico School of Medicine
Physician Assistant Program
Family & Community Medicine

MSC 09 5040, 1 University of New Mexico
Albuquerque, NM
87131-0001
Phone: (505) 272-9678
http://hsc.unm.edu/SOM/fcm/pap/

UNIVERSITY OF ST. FRANCIS

Physician Assistant Program
4401 Silver Avenue, SE, Suite B
Albuquerque, NM
87108
Phone: (888) 446-4657
http://www1.stfrancis.edu/content/conah/pa/

NEVADA

Touro University, Nevada
Physician Assistant Program
College of Osteopathic Medicine
874 American Pacific Drive
Henderson, NV
89014
Phone: (702) 777-1770
http://en.wikipedia.org/wiki/Physician_Assistant

NEW YORK

Albany Medical College
Physician Assistant Program
Center for Physician Assistant Studies
47 New Scotland Avenue, Mail Code 4
Albany, NY

12208-3412
Phone: (518) 262-5251
http://www.amc.edu/Academic/PhysicianAssistant/index.html

CUNY YORK COLLEGE

Physician Assistant Program
94-20 Guy Brewer Blvd, Room 112 SC
Jamaica, NY
11451
Phone: (718) 262-2823
http://york.cuny.edu/academics/departments/health-professions/
program-courses/physician-assistant-program
D'Youville College
Physician Assistant Program
320 Porter Avenue
Buffalo, NY
14201
Phone: (716) 829-7713
http://www.dyc.edu/academics/physician_assistant/index.asp

DAEMEN COLLEGE

Physician Assistant Department
4380 Main Street
Amherst, NY
14226-3592
Phone: (800) 462-7652
http://www.daemen.edu/academics/physician_assistant/

HOFSTRA UNIVERSITY

Physician Assistant Studies Program
113 Monroe Lecture Hall

127 Hofstra University
Hempstead, NY
11549
Phone: (516) 463-4074
http://www.hofstra.edu/Academics/Colleges/HCLAS/PAP/

LE MOYNE COLLEGE

Physician Assistant Program
Department of Biology
1419 Salt Springs Road
Syracuse, NY
13214-1399
Phone: (315) 445-4745
http://www.lemoyne.edu/tabid/654/Default.aspx

LONG ISLAND UNIVERSITY

Physician Assistant Program
121 DeKalb Avenue
Brooklyn, NY
11201
Phone: (718) 260-2780
http://www.brooklyn.liu.edu/health/bsphyass.html

MERCY COLLEGE

Graduate Program in Physician Assistant Studies
1200 Waters Place
Bronx, NY
10461
Phone: (914) 674-7635
https://contest.mercy.edu/pages/865.asp

NEW YORK INSTITUTE OF TECHNOLOGY

Physician Assistant Program
Riland Building, Suite 352—Northern Blvd
Old Westbury, NY
11568-8000
Phone: (516) 686-3881
http://www.nyit.edu/physician_assistant_studies/

PACE UNIVERSITY-LENOX HILL HOSPITAL

Physician Assistant Program
One Pace Plaza, Room Y-31
New York, NY
10038
Phone: (212) 346-1357
http://www.pace.edu/page.cfm?doc_id=6594

ROCHESTER INSTITUTE OF TECHNOLOGY

Physician Assistant Program
85 Lomb Memorial Drive
Rochester, NY
14623-5603
Phone: (584) 475-2978
http://www.rit.edu/cos/medical/physician_assistant.html

SUNY/DOWNSTATE MEDICAL CENTER

Physician Assistant Program
Health Science Center
450 Clarkson Avenue—Box 1222
Brooklyn, NY

11203
Phone: (718) 270-2324) 5
http://www.downstate.edu/pa/

ST. JOHN'S UNIVERSITY

Physician Assistant Education Program
Dr. Andrew Bartilucci Center
175-05 Horace Harding Expressway
Fresh Meadows, NY
11365
Phone: (718) 990-8417
http://www.stjohns.edu/admission/undergraduate/learnmore/

PHYSASSIST

Stony Brook University, SUNY
Physician Assistant Program
School of Health Technology & Management
SHTM—HSC, L2-424
Stony Brook, NY
11794-8202
Phone: (631) 444-3190 ext. 6
http://www.hsc.stonybrook.edu/shtm/pa/index.cfm

SOPHIE DAVIS SCHOOL OF BIOMEDICAL EDUCATION

CUNY Medical School
Harlem Hospital Center
138th Street and Convent Ave, Harris Hall, Suite G15
New York, NY
10031
Phone: (212) 650-7745
http://www1.ccny.cuny.edu/prospective/med/programs/
paprogram.cfm

TOURO COLLEGE

Physician Assistant Program
School of Health Sciences
1700 Union Blvd.
Bay Shore, NY
11706
Phone: (631) 665-1600
http://www.touro.edu/shs/pa.asp

TOURO COLLEGE, MANHATTAN CAMPUS

Physician Assistant Program
School of Health Sciences
27-33 West 23rd Street
New York, NY
10010
Phone: (212) 463-0400, ext. 792
http://www.touro.edu/shs/pany/

WAGNER COLLEGE/STATEN ISLAND UNIVERSITY HOSPITAL

Physician Assistant Program
One Campus Road
Staten Island, NY
10301
Phone: (718) 420-4142 or 4151
http://www.wagner.edu/departments/pa_program/3yrPA

WEILL CORNELL MEDICAL COLLEGE

Physician Assistant Program (A Surgical Focus)
575 Lexington Avenue, Suite 600

New York, NY
10022
Phone: (646) 962-7277
http://www.med.cornell.edu/education/programs/phy_ass.html

OHIO

Cuyahoga Community College
Physician Assistant Program
11000 Pleasant Valley Road
Parma, OH
44130
Phone: (216) 987-5363
http://www.tri-c.edu/programs/physicianassistant/Pages/
default.aspx

KETTERING COLLEGE OF MEDICAL ARTS

Physician Assistant Program
3737 Southern Boulevard
Kettering, OH
45429
Phone: (937) 296-7238
http://www.kcma.edu/academics/pa/index.html

MARIETTA COLLEGE

Physician Assistant Program
215 Fifth Street
Marietta, OH
45750
Phone: (740) 376-4458
http://www.marietta.edu/~paprog/

MOUNT UNION COLLEGE

Physician Assistant Program
1972 Clark Avenue
Alliance, OH
44601
Phone: (800) 334-6682
http://www2.muc.edu/Newsroom/February08/
physician_assistant_master_program_first_since_1912.aspx

UNIVERSITY OF FINDLAY

Physician Assistant Program
1000 North Main Street
Findlay, OH
45840-3695
Phone: (419) 434-4529
http://www.findlay.edu/academics/colleges/cohp/
academicprograms/undergraduate/PHAS/default.htm

UNIVERSITY OF TOLEDO

Physician Assistant Program
School of Allied Health
3015 Arlington Avenue
Toledo, OH
43614-5803
Phone: (419) 383-5408
http://www.utoledo.edu/hshs/pa/index.html

OKLAHOMA

University of Oklahoma
Physician Assistant Program

Health Sciences Center
PO Box 26901
Oklahoma City, OK
73190
Phone: (405) 271-2058
http://www.okpa.org/Default.aspx?alias=www.okpa.org/paprogram

UNIVERSITY OF OKLAHOMA, TULSA

Physician Assistant Program
4502 E. 41st Street
Tulsa, OK
74135-2512
Phone: (918) 619-4760
http://tulsa.ou.edu/pa/

OREGON

Oregon Health Sciences University
Physician Assistant Program
3181 SW Sam Jackson Park Road
GH219
Portland, OR
97239-3098
Phone: (503) 494-1484
http://www.ohsu.edu/xd/education/schools/school-of-medicine/
academic-programs/physician-assistant/index.cfm

PACIFIC UNIVERSITY

Physician Assistant Program
School of Physician Assistant Studies
2043 College Way

Forest Grove, OR
97116
Phone: (503) 352-2898
http://www.pacificu.edu/pa/

PENNSYLVANIA

Arcadia University
Physician Assistant Program
Brubaker Hall, Health Science Center
450 South Easton Road
Glenside, PA
19038
Phone: (215) 572-2082
http://www.arcadia.edu/academic/default.aspx?id=425

CHATHAM COLLEGE

Physician Assistant Program
Woodland Road
Pittsburgh, PA
15232
Phone: (412) 365-1412
http://www.chatham.edu/departments/healthmgmt/graduate/pa/

DESALES UNIVERSITY

Physician Assistant Program
2755 Station Avenue
Center Valley, PA
18034-9568
Phone: (610) 282-1100 x1415
http://www.desales.edu/physician_assistant_studies_degree_pa.aspx

DREXEL UNIVERSITY HAHNEMANN

Physician Assistant Program
College of Nursing and Health Professions
1505 Race Street, 8th Floor, MS 504
Philadelphia, PA
19102-1192
Phone: (215) 762-7135
http://www.drexel.edu/cnhp/physician_assistant/masters_about.asp

DUQUESNE UNIVERSITY

Physician Assistant Program
John G. Rangos, Sr., School of Health Sciences
323 Health Sciences Building
Pittsburgh, PA
15282
http://www.healthsciences.duq.edu/pa/pahome.html

GANNON UNIVERSITY

Physician Assistant Program
109 University Square
Erie, PA
16541-0001
Phone: (814) 871-7474
http://www.gannon.edu/PROGRAMS/UNDER/phyasst.asp

KING'S COLLEGE

Physician Assistant Program
133 North River Street
Wilkes-Barre, PA
18711

Phone: (570) 208-5853
www.kings.edu/paprog

LOCK HAVEN UNIVERSITY OF PENNSYLVANIA

Physician Assistant Program
Lock Haven, PA
17745
Phone: (570) 893-2541
http://gradprograms.lhup.edu/pa/

MARYWOOD UNIVERSITY

Physician Assistant Program
2300 Adams Avenue
Scranton, PA
18509
Phone: (570) 348-6298
http://www.marywood.edu/pa-program/

PENNSYLVANIA COLLEGE OF OPTOMETRY

Physician Assistant Program
8360 Old York Road
Elkins Park, PA
19027
Phone: (215) 780-1515
http://www.salus.edu/images/pa/health_science.html

PENNSYLVANIA COLLEGE OF TECHNOLOGY

Physician Assistant Program
DIF #123

One College Avenue
Williamsport, PA
17701-5799
Phone: (570) 327-4779
http://www.pct.edu/

PHILADELPHIA COLLEGE OF OSTEOPATHIC MEDICINE

Department of Physician Assistant Studies
4190 City Avenue, Rowland Hall
Philadelphia, PA
19131
Phone: (215) 871-6772
http://www.pcom.edu/academic_programs/aca_pa/degree_
programs_physician_assi/degree_programs_physician_assi.html

PHILADELPHIA UNIVERSITY

Physician Assistant Program
School House Lane & Henry Avenue
Philadelphia, PA
19144
Phone: (215) 951-2908
http://www.philau.edu/PAProgram/

SAINT FRANCIS UNIVERSITY

Department of Physician Assistant Sciences
PO Box 600
Loretto, PA
15940-0600
Phone: (814) 472-3020
http://www.francis.edu/MPAShome.htm

SETON HILL UNIVERSITY

Physician Assistant Program
Seton Hill Drive
Greensburg, PA
15601
Phone: (724) 838-4283
http://www.setonhill.edu/academics/pa/index.cfm

SOUTH CAROLINA

Medical University of South Carolina
Physician Assistant Program
College of Health Professions
PO Box 250856
Charleston, SC
29425
Phone: (843) 792-1913
http://www.musc.edu/chp/pa/

SOUTH DAKOTA

University of South Dakota
Physician Assistant Studies Program
School of Medicine
414 East Clark Street
Vermillion, SD
57069-2390
Phone: (605) 677-5128
http://www.usd.edu/pa/

TENNESSEE

Bethel College
Physician Assistant Program

325 Cherry Avenue, Box 329
McKenzie, TN
38201
Phone: (731) 352-5708
http://www.bethel-college.edu/bethelpa/index.htm

LINCOLN MEMORIAL UNIVERSITY—DEBUSK COLLEGE OF OSTEOPATHIC MEDICINE

Physician Assistant Program
6965 Cumberland Gap Parkway
Harrogate, TN
37752
http://www.lmunet.edu/DCOM/pa/index.htm

SOUTH COLLEGE

Master of Health Science—Physician Assistant Program
3904 Lonas Drive
Knoxville, TN
37909
Phone: (865) 251-1800
http://www.southcollegetn.edu/masters/physician-assistant/

TREVECCA NAZARENE UNIVERSITY

Physician Assistant Program
333 Murfreesboro Road
Nashville, TN
37210-2877
Phone: (615) 248-1225
http://www.trevecca.edu/pa

TEXAS

Baylor College of Medicine
Physician Assistant Program
Room 107 BTXX, One Baylor Plaza
Houston, TX
77030-3498
Phone: (713) 798-4842
http://www.bcm.edu/pap/

TEXAS TECH UNIVERSITY HEALTH SCIENCES CENTER

School of Allied Health, Department of Diagnostic & Primary Care
Physician Assistant Program
3600 North Garfield
Midland, TX
79705
Phone: (915) 620-9905
http://www.ttuhsc.edu/sah/mpa/

UNIVERSITY OF TEXAS, PAN AMERICAN

Physician Assistant Studies Program
1201 W. University Drive
Edinburg, TX
78539
Phone: (956) 381-2298
http://portal.utpa.edu/utpa_main/daa_home/hshs_home/pasp_home

UNIVERSITY OF TEXAS HEALTH SCIENCE CENTER AT SAN ANTONIO

Physician Assistant Program
Department of Physician Assistant Studies

7703 Floyd Curl Drive, MC 6249
San Antonio, TX
78229-3900
Phone: (210) 567-8811
http://www.uthscsa.edu/shp/pa/

UNIVERSITY OF TEXAS MEDICAL BRANCH

Physician Assistant Program
School of Allied Health Services
301 University Boulevard
Galveston, TX
77555-1145
Phone: (409) 772-3046
http://www.sahs.utmb.edu/PAS/

UNIVERSITY OF NORTH TEXAS

Physician Assistant Studies
Health Science Center at Fort Worth
3500 Camp Bowie Boulevard
Fort Worth, TX
76107-2699
Phone: (817) 735-2301
http://www.hsc.unt.edu/education/PASP/

UNIVERSITY OF TEXAS, SOUTHWESTERN MEDICAL CENTER AT DALLAS

Physician Assistant Program
6011 Harry Hines Boulevard
Dallas, TX
75390-9090

Phone: (214) 648-1701
http://www.utsouthwestern.edu/utsw/cda/dept48945/files/54102.html

UTAH

University of Utah
Physician Assistant Program
375 Chipeta Way
Salt Lake City, UT
84108
Phone: (801) 581-7766
http://web.utah.edu/upap/

VIRGINIA

Eastern Virginia Medical School
Physician Assistant Program
700 West Olney Road, Suite 1110
PO Box 1980
Norfolk, VA
23501-1980
Phone: (757) 446-7158
http://www.evms.edu/hlthprof/mpa/

JAMES MADISON UNIVERSITY

Physician Assistant Program
Dept of Health Sciences, MSC 4301
Harrisonburg, VA
22807
Phone: (540) 568-2395
http://www.jmu.edu/healthsci/paweb/

JEFFERSON COLLEGE OF HEALTH SCIENCES

Physician Assistant Program
920 S. Jefferson Street
Roanoke, VA
24016
Phone: (540) 985-4016
    http://www.jchs.edu/page.php/prmID/77

SHENANDOAH UNIVERSITY

Division of Physician Assistant Studies
1460 University Drive
Winchester, VA
22601
Phone: (540) 542-6208
http://www.su.edu/

WASHINGTON

University of Washington
MEDEX Northwest
Physician Assistant Program
4311 11th Ave NE, Suite 200
Seattle, WA
98105-4608
Phone: (206) 616-4001
http://www.washington.edu/medicine/som/depts/medex/

WISCONSIN

Marquette University
Department of Physician Assistant Studies
College of Health Sciences

1700 Building—PO Box 1881
Milwaukee, WI
53201-1881
Phone: (414) 288-5688
http://www.marquette.edu/chs/pa/index.shtml

UNIVERSITY OF WISCONSIN, LACROSSE; GUNDERSON LUTHERAN MEDICAL

Foundation; Mayo School of Health-Related Sciences
Physician Assistant Program
1725 State Street, 4031 Health Science Center
LaCrosse, WI
54601-3767
Phone: (608) 785-8470
http://perth.uwlax.edu/pastudies/

UNIVERSITY OF WISCONSIN, MADISON

Physician Assistant Program
Room 1278 Health Sciences Learning Center
750 Highland Avenue
Madison, WI
53705
Phone: (608) 263-5620
http://www.physicianassistant.wisc.edu/

WEST VIRGINIA

Alderson Broaddus College
Physician Assistant Department
PO Box 2036
Philippi, WV
26416

Phone: (304) 457-6283
http://www.ab.edu/academics/degrees/physician_assistant_studies

MOUNTAIN STATE UNIVERSITY

Physician Assistant Program
609 South Kanawha Street, PO Box 9003
Beckley, WV
25802-9003
Phone: (304) 253-7351
http://www.mountainstate.edu/majors/onlinecatalogs/graduate/programs/
PhysiciansAssistant.aspx

Get Into the PA School of Your Choice

Getting accepted to PA school is a highly competitive process. If you want to maximize your chances for success, visit www.AndrewRodican.com and sign up for a coaching package now!

Andrew Rodican, PA-C will personally help you:

- Navigate the CASPA application process
- Write a "killer" essay that will make an emotional connection with the admissions committee and get you an interview
- "Ace" the PA school interview and get accepted

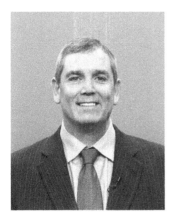

Andrew J. Rodican, PA-C is the author of *The Ultimate Guide to Getting into Physician Assistant School* and *How to "Ace" the Physician Assistant School Interview.*